Drugs
in
Sport

Drugs in Sport

Edited by

D. R. MOTTRAM

B Pharm, PhD, MPS

Human Kinetics Books
CHAMPAIGN, ILLINOIS

First published in 1988 by E. & F. N. Spon Ltd
11 New Fetter Lane, London EC4P 4EE
Published in the USA by
Human Kinetics Publishers, Inc.
Box 5076, Champaign, IL 61820

Set in 10/12 pt Ehrhardt by Scarborough Typesetting Services

Printed in Great Britain by St Edmundsbury Press Ltd, Bury St.
Edmunds, Suffolk

ISBN 0 87322 222 9

Contents

Contributors

D. J. Armstrong, BSc, PhD

P. N. C. Elliott, BSc, PhD

A. J. George, BSc, LI Biol, PhD

D. R. Mottram, B Pharm, PhD, MPS

T. Reilly, BA, Dip PE, MSc, PhD, MI Biol, F Erg S

All contributors are currently affiliated to

School of Health Sciences,
Liverpool Polytechnic,
Liverpool, UK.

Foreword

Sport is an integral part of a healthy lifestyle in today's society. Yet society has come to rely increasingly upon drugs to treat illness, ease pain and to maintain life. Sadly, we are all too aware of the abuse of drugs in sport to enhance performance. This is the very antithesis of sport and of the Olympic ideal.

Our knowledge of sporting performance has developed to an advanced level, to that of a technical science. Coaching and training can be improved with the application of the principles of sports science, whilst sports medicine expertise can be vital to the maintenance of health and to assist with the treatment of injuries. However, the place of drugs in the training regime and competitive programme is surrounded by controversy and misunderstanding.

I welcome the publication of this book as a step in the right direction. I believe it takes a balanced, informative approach to the use and abuse of drugs in sport. The concern is not simply about ethical issues but also for the health of the competitor.

SEBASTIAN COE

Postscript – the 1988 Olympic Games

The 1988 Olympic Games in Seoul will be remembered as much for events in the drug testing laboratories as for achievements in the sporting arena.

Several competitors from widely differing sporting disciplines were found to have taken banned substances when subjected to the routine testing procedures at the Games. The types of drugs which had been taken included central stimulants such as caffeine and pemoline, beta blockers such as propanolol, sympathomimetics such as pseudo-ephedrine, diuretics such as frusemide and, most notoriously, the anabolic steroid stanozolol.

Of those competitors found to have taken banned substances, ten were disqualified, which is two fewer than in the Los Angeles Olympics of 1984 and only one more than the 1980 Games in Moscow. The pre-Games reports of widespread drug misuse appear to have been unfounded. It could be argued that competitors stopped taking their drugs prior to the Games in Seoul in order to avoid detection. However, most classes of banned substances, with the major exception of the anabolic steroids, are only likely to have an effect at the time of competition. If drug taking was temporarily halted during the Games then the performances recorded in most events suggest that either very few competitors had used drugs previously to enhance performance or that such drugs do not have any significant performance enhancing properties.

In the earlier stages of the Games, reports of positive drug tests attracted little attention from the media even though one or two competitors were stripped of their medals and Olympic titles as a result.

It was not until the Canadian, Ben Johnson, was found to have taken the anabolic steroid stanozolol that the world's interest was focused on the whole question of drug abuse in sport and the implications for both the drug taker and for the future of sport itself.

A number of important conclusions can be drawn from events in Seoul. Firstly, it is clear that the sensitivity and accuracy of the drug testing procedures has reached an extremely high level of sophistication. Even the anabolic steroids and their metabolites, which had hitherto proved difficult to analyse were easily detected.

Secondly, it was surprising that so many competitors were found to have taken banned substances, especially considering the wealth of experience and expertise within the national squads, from which competitors could have sought advice and guidance. The reasons may be manifold. It is clear from statements made by competitors, pundits and commentators that there is still widespread ignorance with regard to the actions, side effects and supposed performance enhancing properties of drugs. Some competitors may have thrown caution to the wind in an attempt to gain maximum advantage over their fellow competitors. On the other hand some competitors may have paid the penalty of making a miscalculation in their attempt to avoid detection. This latter proposal may be related to the previously discussed issue of the more sophisticated testing procedures currently available.

Thirdly, the world's attention has now been firmly drawn to the problem of drug abuse in sport. It appeared from the scant coverage given to incedences involving drugs in sport both before and during the early stages of the Seoul Olympics that drug taking had somehow become an accepted, if not condoned, part of sport. The involvement of a top athlete like Ben Johnson has at least generated wide media attention and profound discussion of the topic. What does still seem surprising to the author is that in all the ensuing discussion none of those involved appeared to question whether the drugs being taken do in fact produce an enhanced performance. Unfortunately there is too little evidence, based on controlled trials and incorporating sound scientific principles, to allow rational conclusions to be drawn on this question. Who is to know whether medal winning athletes, stripped of their titles, would have won medals without recourse to drugs. Likewise, how many competitors who were also taking drugs were not in contention for medals? It is to be hoped that those pundits who espouse the use of drugs by athletes and consider that the testing for drugs should be abolished, do not gain support from public opinion. The consequences for sport in general and for young participants in particular would be devastating.

Finally, the question of amateurism versus professionalism in sport must be raised. It is clear from the Seoul Olympics that the IOC are moving ever closer to an 'open' Olympics with the admission of professional sportsmen and women in sports such as tennis and soccer and, considering the large sums of money which are paid to top performers in athletics and other sports, with the inevitable increase in sponsorship for successful competitors the incentive to win will be immense. This will undoubtedly encourage performers to accept whatever means are available to them in an attempt to attain supremity in their chosen sport. With the burgeoning supply network of drugs many performers will be tempted to experiment. It is to be hoped that events in the 1988 Olympic Games in Seoul will cause sportsmen and women to think very carefully about the consequences of taking drugs, either deliberately or accidently. It is also to be hoped that with the renewed confidence in the drug testing procedures amply exhibited at Seoul, all national administrators for sport will initiate or step up, as appropriate, programmes of random out-of-season drug testing within their countries so that the 1992 Olympic Games in Barcelona will be memorable more for events on rather than off the field of competition.

DAVID R. MOTTRAM
October 1988

Glossary
of terms

Absorption The process through which a drug passes from its site of administration into the blood.

Addison's disease A disorder caused by degeneration of the adrenal cortex resulting in impairment of sodium reabsorption from the urine.

Adrenal glands The two glands which comprise an outer cortex which produces the mineralocorticoid and glucocorticoid hormones and the inner medulla which produces the hormone adrenaline.

Adrenaline A hormone released from the adrenal medulla under conditions of stress; sometimes referred to as epinephrine.

Adrenoceptors Receptors (subclassified alpha and beta) through which adrenaline, noradrenaline and sympathomimetic drugs exert their effects.

Agonist A drug that interacts with receptors to produce a response in a tissue or organ.

Agranulocytosis The destruction of granulocytes (blood cells) often induced by drugs. The condition responds to treatment by corticosteroids.

Allergy A hypersensitivity reaction in which antibodies are produced in response to food, drugs or environmental antigens (allergens) to which they have previously been exposed.

Anabolic steroid A hormone or drug which produces retention of nitrogen, potassium and phosphate, increases protein synthesis and decreases amino acid breakdown.

Analgesic drug A drug which can relieve pain. Generally they are subclassified as narcotic analgesics, e.g. morphine or non-narcotic analgesics, e.g. aspirin.

Anaphylaxis An immediate hypersensitivity reaction, following administration of a drug or other agent, in an individual who has previously been exposed to the drug and who has produced antibodies to that drug. It is characterized by increased vascular permeability and bronchoconstriction.

Androgen A steroidal drug which promotes the development of male secondary sexual characteristics.

Anorectic agent A drug which suppresses appetite through an action in the central nervous system.

Antagonist drug A drug that occupies receptors without producing a response but prevents the action of an endogenous substance or an agonist drug.

Antihistamine drug An antagonist drug which stops the action of histamine and therefore is used in the treatment of hay fever.

Antihypertensive drug A drug which lowers abnormally high blood pressure.

Anti-inflammatory drug A drug that reduces the symptoms of inflammation and includes glucocorticosteroids and non-steroidal anti-inflammatory drugs, such as aspirin.

Antipyretic drug A drug which can reduce an elevated body temperature.

Antitussive drug A drug which suppresses coughing either by a local soothing effect or by depressing the cough centre in the CNS.

Atherosclerosis The accumulation of lipid deposits such as cholesterol and triacylglycerol on the walls of arteries. These fatty plaques can lead to a narrowing of arteries and therefore ischaemia or can encourage the formation of a thrombus (blood clot).

Atopy The acquisition of sensitivity to various environmental substances, such as pollen and house dust, thereby rendering the individual allergic to those substances.

Atrophy A wasting away or decrease in size of a mature tissue.

Axon A projection of nerve cell bodies which conduct impulses to the target tissue.

Beta blocker An antagonist of the beta group of adrenoceptors with a wide variety of clinical uses, principally in treating angina and hypertension.

Blind or double-blind trial A method for testing the effectiveness of a drug on a group of subjects where the subjects alone (blind) or the subjects and evaluators (double-blind) are prevented from knowing whether the active drug or a placebo has been administered.

Blood–brain barrier The cells of the capillaries in the brain which impede the access of certain substances in the blood from reaching the brain.

Bronchodilator drug A drug which relaxes the smooth muscle in the respiratory tract thereby dilating the airways. Many bronchodilators are agonists on $beta_2$-adrenoceptors.

Capillaries Blood vessels whose walls are a single layer of cells thick, through which water and solutes exchange between the blood and the tissue fluid.

Cardiac output The volume of blood per minute ejected from the left ventricle of the heart.

Cardiac rate The number of times the heart beats each minute. The normal resting heart rate is around 60 beats per minute.

Cardioselective beta blockers Antagonists of beta-adrenoceptors which have a selective action on the beta$_1$-adrenoceptors, a major site of which is the cardiac muscle in the heart.

Chemotaxis Chemical mediated attraction of leucocytes to a site of injury.

Cholinergic neurones Nerve fibres that release acetylcholine from their nerve terminals.

Claudication Pain caused by temporary constriction of blood vessels supplying skeletal muscle.

Coronary heart disease Malfunction of the heart caused by occlusion of the artery supplying the heart muscle.

Coronary occlusion Obstruction of the arteries supplying heart muscle either through vasoconstriction or a mechanical obstruction such as an atheromatous plaque or blood clot.

Cumulation The process by which the blood levels of a drug build up thereby increasing its therapeutic and toxic effects.

Diabetes mellitus A disorder of carbohydrate metabolism, characterized by an increased blood sugar level, caused by decreased insulin activity.

Diuresis Increased output of urine which may be induced by disease or the action of drugs.

Dose regime The amount of drug taken, expressed in terms of the quantity of drug and the frequency at which it is taken.

Drug allergy A reaction to a drug which involves the production of antibodies when first exposed to the drug.

Drug dependence A compulsion to take a drug on a continuous basis both to experience its psychic effects and to avoid the adverse physical effects experienced when the drug is withdrawn.

Drug idiosyncracy A genetically determined abnormal reactivity to a drug.

Drug metabolism The chemical alteration of drug molecules by the body to aid in the detoxification and excretion of the drug.

Electromyography The measurement of muscular contraction using needle electrodes inserted into the muscle.

Electroencephalogram (EEG) A recording of the electrical potential changes occurring in the brain.

Endogenous biochemical A chemical substance such as a hormone or neurotransmitter which is found naturally in the body.

Epinephrine *see* Adrenaline.

Epiphyses The articular end structures of long bones.

European Antidoping Charter for Sport Recommendations adopted by the Committee of Ministers of the Council of Europe in 1984 for the control of drugs in sport.

Generic name The official name of the active drug within a medicine. Different manufacturers of a drug may use their own proprietary or brand name to describe the drug.

Glomeruli The units within the kidney where filtration of the blood takes place.

Glucocorticosteroids Steroid hormones and drugs which affect carbohydrate metabolism more than electrolyte and water balance (cf. mineralocorticoids). They can be used as anti-inflammatory drugs.

Glycogenolysis The breakdown of the storage material, glycogen, into the energy source glucose. Glycogenolysis is a major function of adrenaline.

Hepatic circulation The arteries, capillaries and veins carrying blood to and from the liver.

Hormones Endogenous biochemical messengers that are released from endocrine glands directly into the blood stream. They interact with specific receptors on their target tissues.

Hyperpnoea An increase in the rate and depth of respiration.

Hypertrophy An increase in tissue size due to an increase in the size of functional cells without an increase in the number of cells.

Hypokalaemia A condition in which there is a profound lowering of potassium levels in the extracellular fluid.

Iatrogenic disease Originally the term for physician-caused disease. Now it applies to side effects of drugs caused by inappropriate prescribing or administration of drugs.

Interstitial fluid The water and solute contents of the fluid found between cells of tissues.

Intracellular fluid The water and solute contents of the fluid found within cells.

Ischaemic pain Pain within a tissue induced by reduced blood flow to that tissue.

Isometric contraction Contraction of skeletal (striated) muscle in which the muscle develops tension but does not alter in length.

Isotonic contraction Contraction of skeletal muscle in which the muscle shortens under a constant load, such as occurs during walking, running or lifting.

Kinins Endogenous polypeptides (e.g. kallidin, bradykinin, angiotensin and substance P) which have a marked pharmacological effect on smooth muscle.

Leucocytes White blood cells, comprising several different types with differing functions.

Ligand An atom or molecule (including drugs) that interacts with a larger molecule, at a specific (receptor) site.

Lipolysis The breakdown of fats into free fatty acid.

Mast cells Large cells containing histamine and other substances which are released during allergic responses.

Medicine A preparation containing one or more drugs designed for use as a therapeutic agent.

Metabolite The chemical produced by the metabolic transformation of a drug or other substance.

Mineralocorticoid A steroid hormone which has a selective action on electrolyte and water balance.

Monoamine oxidase A major metabolizing enzyme responsible for the breakdown of monoamines such as adrenaline and noradrenaline.

Mydriasis Contraction of the iris in the eye leading to an increased pupil size.

Myocardium The cardiac muscle which makes up the walls of the heart.

Narcolepsy A disorder characterized by periodic attacks of an overwhelming desire to sleep.

Narcotic analgesic A drug that induces a state of reversible depression of the CNS (narcosis) as well as producing pain relief (analgesia). Most narcotic analgesics are related to morphine.

Nasal decongestant A drug (usually a sympathomimetic) which reduces the mucous secretion in the nasal passages normally by vasoconstriction in the nasal mucosa.

Nebulizer therapy A method of drug administration in which the drug dissolved in a solution, is vaporized and the vapour inhaled. This method is primarily used for bronchodilator drugs.

Necrosis Tissue death.

Neurotransmitter A biochemical agent released from nerve endings to transmit a response to another cell.

Non-steroidal anti-inflammatory drug A drug such as asprin or indomethacin the structure of which is not based on a steroid nucleus and which is able to control the inflammatory response within tissues.

Noradrenaline The neurotransmitter in certain sympathetic and central nerves. Sometimes referred to as norepinephrine.

Oedema Tissue swelling due to accumulation of fluid in the interstitial spaces.

Osteoporosis A condition in which bone tissue becomes demineralized.

Over-the-counter medicines Drugs which can be purchased directly from a pharmacy or drug store without a medical practitioner's prescription.

Paranoia A mental disorder characerized by persistent delusions, particular of persecution or power.

Pepsin A digestive enzyme, secreted in the stomach, that hydrolyses proteins into smaller peptide fractions.

Phagocytosis The ingestion of bacteria or other foreign particles by cells, usually a type of white blood cell.

Pharmacokinetics A study of the absorption, distribution and excretion of drugs using mathematical parameters to measure time courses.

Pharmacology The study of the modes of action, uses and side effects of drugs.

Placebo A substance which is pharmacologically inactive and which is usually used to compare the effects with an active drug in blind or double-blind trials.

Plasma proteins Proteins (albumin and globulins) which circulate in the plasma of blood. Many drugs are capable of binding to these proteins thereby reducing their availability as therapeutic agents.

Prepubertal male A male who has not yet reached the age at which he is capable of adult sexual functions.

Prescription only medicine A therapeutic agent which can only be obtained on the written authority (prescription) of a medical or dental practitioner.

Prostaglandins A group of chemical agents found in the body and which have a wide variety of actions, some of which are involved in inflammation.

Psychomotor stimulant drug A drug which can reduce fatigue and elevate mood. They are also referred to as psychostimulants, psychoanaleptics, psychoactivators and psychotonics.

Pulmonary emphysema A chronic lung disease in which the walls of adjacent alveoli and bronchioles degenerate forming cavities in the lung tissue.

Purulent secretion A secretion (e.g. nasal) containing a bacterial infection.

Receptor An area on a macromolecule through which endogenous bio-chemicals or drugs can interact to produce a cellular response.

Respiratory quotient A parameter used to indicate the nutrient molecules being metabolized within the body. It can be determined by dividing the amount of carbon dioxide produced by the amount of oxygen consumed. On a balanced diet the respiratory quotient should approximate to 0.85.

Re-uptake The mechanism by which neurotransmitters, released from nerve terminals, are taken back into the nerve ending for storage and re-release.

Rheumatic fever Damage to valves of the heart caused by a streptococcal bacterial infection. It is an autoimmune response to the streptococcal toxin.

Rheumatoid arthritis An autoimmune disease principally affecting joints, characterized by pain, inflammation and stiffness.

Rhinitis Inflammation of the mucous membrane within the nose resulting in increased mucous secretion. Rhinitis may be caused by infection or an allergic response.

Salicylates Drugs that are chemically related to salicylic acid. They possess anti-inflammatory, antipyretic and analgesic activity.

Sedative drug A drug which can calm an anxious person without inducing sleep.

Selectivity The ability of a drug to exert a greater effect on a particular population of receptors due to its chemical structure. This property reduces the incidence of side effects.

Serotonin A neurotransmitter substance, also known as 5-hydroxytryptamine.

Spermatogenesis The production of sperm cells from spermatogonia or germ cells within the seminiferous tubules of the testes.

Stroke volume The amount of blood pumped by the ventricles with each beat of the heart.

Sympathomimetic drug A drug which mimics some or all of the effects produced by stimulation of the sympathetic nervous system. The effects it produces depends upon the adrenoceptors through which it interacts.

Glossary of terms   **xvii**

Synapse The narrow gap between the nerve terminal and its target cell into which the neurotransmitter is released.

Tachycardia A rate of beating of the heart above the normal rate.

Tachyphylaxis A rapid decrease in the effect of a drug as the dosage is repeated. It is probably caused by desensitization of receptors.

Therapeutic effect The desired response of a drug taken to treat or cure a disease.

Tolerance The effect whereby increasing doses of a drug have to be given to maintain the desired effect.

Urticaria A localized rash on the skin, usually due to an allergic reaction.

Vascular permeability The passage of fluid and solutes across the membranes of blood vessels.

Vasoconstriction The reduction in the diameter of blood vessels produced by contraction of the smooth muscle in the walls.

Vasodilation Relaxation of vascular smooth muscle leading to an increase in the diameter of blood vessels resulting in a fall in blood pressure.

Withdrawal syndrome The physical response of an individual who is deprived of a drug to which he or she had become physically dependent.

Introduction – Drugs and their use in sport

D. R. MOTTRAM

Historical perspective

The extensive use of medicinal products for the alleviation of the symptoms of disease can be traced back to the Greek physician, Galen, in the third century BC. Interestingly, it was Galen who reported that ancient Greek athletes used stimulants to enhance their physical performance. Up to the middle of this century there has been little documentary evidence available to substantiate the hypothesis that drugs have been used in sport. Periodic reports describing the use by athletes of caffeine, strychnine, ether and alcohol, appeared between the middle of the nineteenth century and the advent of the Second World War. Perhaps the dearth of evidence for the abuse of drugs in sport merely reflects the paucity in the number of therapeutic agents available over this period, coupled with the low potency attributable to these drugs when compared with today's powerful agents. Around the time of the Second World War, the development of amphetamine-like central stimulant drugs reached its peak. These drugs were administered to combat troops in order to enhance their mental awareness and to delay the onset of fatigue. Not surprisingly, in the 1940s and 1950s, amphetamines became the drugs of choice for athletes, particularly in sports such as cycling, where these drug effects were perceived to be beneficial in enhancing sporting performance.

The widespread use of drugs in sport, however, began in the 1960s. This phenomenon must be seen in parallel with two other factors. Firstly, the sixties heralded a more liberal approach to experimentation in drug taking particularly amongst the followers of pop music.

Secondly, and of far greater significance, a 'pharmacological revolution' began in the sixties. The search for more potent, more selective and less toxic drugs, resulted in a vast array of powerful agents capable of altering many biochemical, physiological and psychological functions of the body. Not surprisingly some athletes saw, in these chemical agents, a means of enhancing performance beyond anything that they could achieve by hard work and rigorous training. These athletes felt that they could simply select the most specific drugs to meet their particular needs for improving performance.

Reports of the misuse of drugs in sport were widespread, particularly at the time of the 1964 Olympic Games in Tokyo. Pressure for action at national and international level became intense. The first legislation to combat drug abuse in sport was introduced, by the French, in 1963 followed by the Belgian government two years later. The International Olympic Committee's Medical Commission was established in 1967 with drug misuse as one of its primary responsibilities. Drug testing of Olympic athletes began in the 1968 Olympic Games in Mexico City.

Over the last 20 years, random testing of sportsmen and sportswomen has become a routine procedure practised not only at major national and international events but also during competitions organised by most international sporting federations. Laboratories for the screening and analysis of drugs have been set up, with systems for accreditation of such laboratories, to guarantee the highest possible standards of procedure.

In no way can it be claimed that drug misuse in sport has been abolished by these measures, but the increasing vigilance of those who administer sport, along with the increasing sophistication of the methods for detection of drugs, has gone a long way in curtailing the expansion of this illegal method of performance enhancement.

What are drugs?

DRUGS AND THEIR TARGETS

Drugs are chemical substances which, by interaction can alter the biochemical systems of the body. The branch of science investigating drug action is known as pharmacology. These interactions may be mediated through a variety of target tissues within the body. For example, effects on cardiac muscle can lead to an increase in the force and rate of beating of the heart; stimulation of nerve endings in the central nervous system can produce changes in mood and behaviour; interaction with metabolic processes can be used in the treatment of disorders such as diabetes.

It is important to remember that drugs are designed to rectify imbalances of biochemical systems which have been induced by disease. They are not primarily designed to affect biochemical systems in healthy subjects. Therefore the use of drugs to bring about a physiological response that may enhance performance in sport may be totally inappropriate.

The majority of drugs are produced through chemical synthesis though some drugs are still derived from natural sources, for example, the morphine group of drugs is extracted from the fruiting head of the opium poppy.

Ideally a drug should interact with a single target to produce the desired effect within the body. However, all drugs possess varying degrees of side effects, largely dependent on the extent to which they interact with sites other than their primary target. During their development drugs undergo a rigorous appraisal in an endeavour to achieve maximum selectivity. The aim of selectivity is to increase the drug's ability to interact with those sites responsible for inducing the desired therapeutic effect whilst reducing the drug's secondary target sites which are responsible for producing its side effects.

The sites through which most drug molecules interact are known as receptors. These receptors are normally specific areas within the large macromolecules that make up the structure of cells. They may be located on structures within the cell, such as the nucleus, but most receptor sites are found on the cell membranes. Receptors are present within cells in order that naturally occurring substances, such as neurotransmitters, can induce their biochemical and physiological functions within the body. Neurotransmitters are endogenous chemicals which are released from nerve endings when those nerves are stimulated. Following release they can interact with receptors on other nerves to stimulate further neurological pathways or they may interact with receptors present on muscle cells thereby inducing the muscle to contract or relax.

This interaction between a chemical (ligand) and a receptor is the first step in a series of events which eventually leads to the effect produced. The ligand–receptor interaction can therefore be thought of as a trigger mechanism.

There are many different receptor sites within the body each of which possesses its own specific arrangement of recognition sites. Drugs are designed to interact with the recognition sites of particular receptors thereby inducing an effect in the tissue within which the receptors lie. The more closely a drug can fit into its recognition site the greater the triggering response and therefore the greater the potency of the drug on that tissue. In designing drugs it is sometimes necessary to sacrifice some degree of potency on the target receptor site in order to decrease the drug's ability to interact on other receptors. An imbalance towards the therapeutic effect and away from the side effects is thereby achieved, thus producing a greater degree of selectivity.

AGONISTS AND ANTAGONISTS

A drug which mimics the action of an endogenous biochemical substance is said to be an agonist. Other drugs used in therapeutics are known as antagonists. They also have the ability to interact with receptor sites but, unlike agonists, they do not trigger the series of events leading to a response. Their pharmacological effect is produced by preventing the body's own biochemical agents from interacting with the receptors and therefore inhibiting particular biochemical and physiological processes. A typical example of this can be seen with the group of drugs known as the beta blockers. They exert their pharmacological and therapeutic effects by occupying beta receptors without stimulating a response but, by so doing, prevent the neurotransmitter, noradrenaline, and the hormone, adrenaline, from interacting with these receptors. One of the physiological functions mediated by noradrenaline and adrenaline through beta receptors is to increase heart rate in response to exercise or stress, therefore the administration of a beta blocker antagonizes this effect thereby maintaining a lower heart rate under stress conditions.

The principle of drug selectivity applies to both agonists and antagonists in their design as therapeutic agents. Research into drug–receptor interactions has led to a greater understanding of receptor structure and function and the original concepts of receptors have had to be modified. Consequently, there are many examples of subclassifications of receptor populations allowing for even greater degrees of drug selectivity.

EVALUATION OF DRUG ACTION

To establish the effectiveness of a drug it is important to be able to

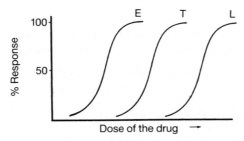

Figure 1 The dose–response relationships for a drug. The three curves represent the dose range over which the drug produces its therapeutic effect (E), toxic effect (T) and lethal effect (L).

quantify its activity. The response to a drug is dependent upon the amount taken. If these two parameters are evaluated then a dose–response relationship for the drug is obtained. The response can be expressed as a percentage of the maximum response obtainable. The dose–response relationship may be plotted graphically (Figure 1). Over the central part of the dose–response curve a linear relationship exists. In the middle of this linear part of the curve lies the 50% response mark, a useful parameter in the evaluation of a drug. The response to a drug can be measured in a variety of ways but there are three important characteristics of response which can be measured and used to evaluate the effectiveness of a drug. The three components are: therapeutic effect, toxic effect and lethality. All drugs exhibit these three components over particular ranges of dosage. The third component is the easiest to define as there is a finite response to be measured, namely, death. The first two components are more difficult to evaluate. The therapeutic effect may be, for example, the alleviation of pain, a response with an ill-defined cut-off point since each individual person will experience a different threshold of tolerance to pain. Therefore widely differing doses of pain killers may be required for different individuals. The toxic effect may be one of several toxic side effects associated with a particular drug. Each one of these side effects may be of greater or lesser clinical significance to the well-being of the patient.

Figure 1 shows the dose–response relationships for the three component parts outlined above. It can be readily visualized that the clinical usefulness of a particular drug will be dependent upon how far apart these three curves are on the dose axis. A drug which exerts its therapeutic effect at low concentrations but which requires much higher concentrations before toxicity appears can be said to be safe. An expression known as the therapeutic index has been used to quantify this principle. The therapeutic index (TI) can be defined as:

$$TI = \frac{\text{Maximum tolerated dose}}{\text{Minimum effective dose}}$$

which in turn can be quantified as:

$$TI = \frac{TD_{50}}{ED_{50}}$$

where the TD_{50} and ED_{50} represent the doses required to produce the toxic and effective therapeutic responses, respectively, in 50% of a group of subjects.

Theoretically, the higher the TI, the better the drug in clinical terms. However, this definition does not take into account the slope of the dose–response curves, which can vary greatly. Thus, not only are the ED_{50} and TD_{50} values of importance but also the degree of overlap between the curves for therapeutic effect and toxic effect.

It is important to remember that all drugs produce toxic side effects though some of these may be deemed acceptable to a patient when weighed against the beneficial therapeutic effects of the drug. However, no such counter balance exists for individuals taking drugs for non-therapeutic purposes where toxic side effects can only be perceived as detrimental to health.

FACTORS AFFECTING DRUG RESPONSES

For a drug to exert its effect it must reach its site of action. This will involve its passage from the site of administration to the cells of the target tissue or organ. The principal factors which can influence this process are the absorption, distribution, metabolism and elimination of the drug. Consideration of these factors is known as the pharmaco-kinetics of drug action.

Absorption

The absorption of a drug is in part dependent upon its route of administration. Many drugs can be applied topically for a localized response. This may take the form of applying a cream, ointment or

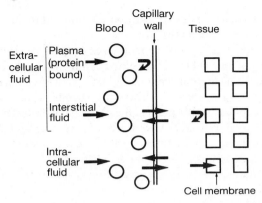

Figure 2 The fluid compartments of the body are 1. plasma (approximately 3 litres); 2. interstitial fluid (9 litres) and 3. intracellular fluid (30 litres). Distribution is dependent on a drug's ability to bind to plasma proteins, and to cross capillary walls or cell membranes.

lotion to an area of skin for treatment of abrasions, lesions, infections or other such dermatological problems. Topical applications may also involve applying drops to the eye or the nose or the inhalation of an aerosol for the topical treatment of respiratory problems.

Most drugs must enter the blood stream in order to reach their site of action and the most common route of administration for this purpose is orally, in either liquid or tablet form. Where a drug is required to act more rapidly, or is susceptible to breakdown in the gastrointestinal tract, the preferred route of administration is by injection. There are a number of routes through which drugs are injected and the main ones are subcutaneous, intramuscular and intravenous.

Distribution

By whatever route the drug is administered a proportion of it will reach the blood stream. Most drugs are then dissolved in the water phase of the blood plasma. Within this phase some of the drug molecules may be bound to proteins and thus may not be freely diffusible out of the plasma. This will affect the amount of drug reaching its target cells. Plasma protein binding is but one factor in the complicated equation of drug distribution. As a general rule the amount of drug reaching the tissue where it exerts its effect is a small part of the total drug concentration in the body. Most of the drug remains in solution within the various fluid compartments of the body (Figure 2).

The principal fluid compartments are: the plasma, the interstitial spaces between the cells and the fluid within the cells of the body (intracellular). These compartments are separated by capillary walls and cell membranes respectively. Therefore, drugs which cannot pass through the capillary wall remain in the plasma. Those drugs which pass through the capillary wall but are unable to cross cell membranes are distributed in the extracellular space and those drugs which permeate all membranes are found within the total body water.

Very few molecules, with the exception of proteins, are unable to cross capillary walls; hence, most drugs, except those which extensively bind to plasma protein, can be found outside the plasma. For a drug to be able to penetrate cell membranes it must be lipid soluble as well as water soluble. The majority of drugs are lipid soluble and are therefore widely distributed throughout the total body water. Drugs which are not lipid soluble are unable to penetrate the cells of the gastrointestinal tract and are therefore poorly absorbed orally. Such drugs must be administered by injection.

An additional obstruction to the passage of drugs occurs at the so-called 'blood–brain barrier' which comprises a layer of cells which covers the capillary walls of the blood vessels supplying the brain. This barrier effectively excludes molecules which are poorly lipid soluble. The blood–brain barrier is an important factor to be considered in designing drugs since a drug's ability to cross this barrier can influence its balance of therapeutic and toxic effects.

Metabolism

The body has a very efficient system for transforming chemicals into safer molecules which can then be excreted by the various routes of elimination. This process is known as metabolism and many drugs which enter the circulation undergo metabolic change.

There are several enzyme systems which are responsible for producing metabolic transformations. These enzymes are principally located in the cells of the liver but may also be found in other cells. They produce simple chemical alteration of the drug molecules by processes such as oxidation, reduction, hydrolysis, acetylation and alkylation.

The consequences of drug metabolism may be seen in a number of ways:

1. An active drug is changed into an inactive compound. This is a common metabolic process and is largely responsible for the termination of the activity of a drug.
2. An active drug can be metabolized into another active compound. The metabolite may have the same pharmacological action as the parent drug or it may differ in terms of higher or lower potency or a different pharmacological effect.
3. An active drug can be changed into a toxic metabolite.
4. An inactive drug can be converted into pharmacologically active metabolites. This mechanism can occasionally be used for beneficial purposes where a drug is susceptible to rapid breakdown before it reaches its site of action. In this case a 'prodrug' can be synthesized which is resistant to breakdown, but which will be metabolized to the active drug on arrival at its target tissue.

Generally speaking, metabolism of drugs results in the conversion of lipid soluble drugs into more water-soluble metabolites. This change affects distribution, in that less lipid soluble compounds are unable to penetrate cell membranes. The kidneys are able to excrete water soluble compounds more readily than lipid soluble molecules since the latter can be reabsorbed in the kidney tubules and therefore re-enter the plasma.

Metabolism is a very important factor in determining a drug's activity since it can alter the drug's intrinsic activity, its distribution and therefore its ability to reach its site of action, and its rate of elimination from the body.

Excretion

There are many routes through which drugs can be eliminated from the body. They may be excreted through salivary glands, sweat glands, pulmonary epithelium and mammary glands. Excretion via the faeces may take place either by passage from the blood into the colon or through secretion with the bile.

The most important route for drug excretion, however, is through the kidneys into the urine. Most drugs and their metabolites are small molecules which are water soluble and as such can be easily filtered through the capillary within the glomeruli of the kidneys. Having been filtered out from the plasma, the molecules may be reabsorbed, to a greater or lesser extent, from the renal tubules. This will depend on their lipid/water partition coefficients, and on whether there is a specific membrane carrier transport system for the particular molecule. The net effect, in all cases, is that a constant fraction of the drug is eliminated at each passage of the blood through the kidney filtration system. The drug and/or its metabolites are then voided with the urine.

Effect of Exercise on Pharmacokinetics

Under most circumstances exercise does not affect the pharmacokinetics of drug action. During severe or prolonged exercise, blood flow within the body will be altered, with a decrease in blood supply to the gastrointestinal tract and to the kidneys. However, there is little documentary evidence to suggest that such changes significantly affect the pharmacokinetics of the majority of drugs.

SIDE EFFECTS OF DRUGS

There are many different receptor sites throughout the body through which drugs can interact and produce pharmacological effects. The same receptor may be found in several different tissues and organs within the body. It is not surprising, therefore, that drugs exhibit a multiplicity of actions. Usually a drug is prescribed for the purposes of producing its most pharmacologically active response, which is its desired or therapeutic effect. Responses other than this are usually unwanted and are referred to as side effects. For example, sufferers from hay fever are frequently prescribed antihistamine drugs whose therapeutic effect is to prevent histamine, which is responsible for many of the symptoms associated with hay fever, from occupying the receptor sites through which it exerts its effect. Therapeutically, antihistamines relieve the symptoms of hay fever principally associated with the respiratory tract and the eyes. However, antihistamines can also cross the blood–brain barrier where they occupy receptors in the central nervous system resulting in a central depressant effect which manifests itself as drowsiness. This is obviously an undesirable side effect of antihistamines since patients receiving these drugs are advized not to drive a vehicle or operate machinery. Under different circumstances, however, this central depressant effect of antihistamines has been turned to a therapeutic use, where such drugs can be administered to calm an excited or feverish child and to promote sleep.

In another example, opiate drugs, such as morphine, have a potent analgesic action which is their primary therapeutic effect. They also produce constipation and respiratory depression as side effects. These side effects of drugs can vary from mild untoward effects which, though unpleasant, can be tolerated, through to effects which are positively deleterious to health and can be described as toxic. It is extremely difficult to draw a line between these two extremes. In general, the distinction between a desirable (therapeutic) effect and a toxic effect is as much quantitative as qualitative and every drug is potentially toxic if administered in high enough doses. *A completely non-toxic drug does not exist.*

Drug toxicity can to a large extent, be predictable. The toxic side effects of drugs are usually well documented as a result of extensive toxicity studies during the development of the drug and from adverse reaction reporting once the drug is on the market. These predictable toxic effects are more pronounced when the drug is taken in overdose. This could occur intentionally (suicide, murder) or accidentally. Accidental overdose may result from children mistaking drugs for sweets; iatrogenic (physician produced) toxicity, resulting from incorrect dosing of patients; patient-induced toxicity when the patient does not comply with the prescribed method of treatment. Accidental toxicity can easily occur with athletes who self-medicate themselves without appreciating the full implications of their actions. The naive philosophy that if one tablet produces a particular desired effect then three tablets must be three times as good frequently applies in these circumstances.

In addition to predictable toxicity, there are a number of ways in which nonpredictable toxicity can occur following the administration of therapeutic or even sub-therapeutic doses of drugs. An example of this is idiosyncrasy where a drug produces an unusual reaction within an individual. This effect is normally genetically determined and is often due to a biochemical deficiency, resulting in the patient's over-reaction to the drug. This may be due to their inability to metabolize the drug.

A second type of nonpredictable toxicity is drug allergy. This is an acquired qualitatively altered reaction of the body to a drug. It differs from normal toxicity to drugs in that the patient will only exhibit the reaction if they have been previously exposed to the drug or a closely related chemical. This initial exposure to the drug, or its metabolite, sensitizes the patient by inducing an allergic response. The drug combines with a protein within the body to produce an antigen, which, in turn, leads to the formation of other proteins called antibodies. This reaction in itself does not induce toxic effects. However, subsequent exposure to the drug will initiate an antigen–antibody reaction. This allergic reaction can manifest itself in a variety of ways. An acute reaction is known as anaphylaxis and normally occurs within one hour of taking the drug. This response frequently involves the respiratory and cardiovascular systems and is often fatal. Subacute allergic reactions usually occur between one and twenty-four hours after the drug is taken and the most common manifestations involve skin reactions, blood dyscrasias, fever and dysfunctions of the respiratory, kidney, liver and cardiovascular systems. Delayed allergic reactions may occur in some cases. This is known as serum sickness syndrome and occurs several days after the drug has been administered.

COMPLEX DRUG REACTIONS

In addition to the side effects associated with drugs there are other complex reactions which may occur. These are particularly likely to happen during long-term usage of a drug or where more than one drug is being taken simultaneously.

The dose regime for a drug is chosen with the objective of maintaining a therapeutic dose level within the body. This regime is determined by two factors: the potency of the drug, which dictates the concentration required at each administration and the rate of metabolism and excretion of the drug, which dictates how frequently the dose has to be taken. If the frequency of administration exceeds the elimination rate of a drug, then that drug will cumulate in the body thereby increasing the likelihood of toxicity reactions. The reason for a slow elimination may be related to a slow metabolism, a strong tendency to plasma protein binding or an inhibition of excretion such as occurs in patients with kidney disease.

Sometimes the drug itself is not cumulative, but its effect is. An example of this can be seen when a drug inhibits an enzyme system. The drug may be present in the body for only a short period of time but the cumulative inhibition of the enzyme, each time the drug is taken, may exceed the rate at which the enzyme system can be regenerated for normal function.

The opposite response to cumulation is seen in patients with drug resistance. This drug resistance may be genetically inherited or acquired. The former type of resistance is not common in humans, though it is an increasing problem in antibacterial therapy where pathogenic microbes can develop genetic changes in their structure or biochemistry which renders them resistant to antibiotic drugs. Acquired resistance to drugs, also known as tolerance, can develop with repeated administration of a drug. Where tolerance occurs, more drug is needed to produce the same pharmacological response. There are several mechanisms responsible for acquired resistance.

Decreased intestinal absorption can develop with repeated use of a drug. It has been observed that chronic alcoholics absorb less alcohol from the gastrointestinal tract. Increased elimination of drugs, either through enhanced metabolism or a more rapid excretion rate, can induce tolerance. In the case of increased metabolism, chemically related substances may induce cross tolerance to each other.

A very rapidly developing tolerance is known as tachyphylaxis and is seen when a drug is repeatedly administered with a decreasing response to each administration. This is usually caused by a slow rate of detachment of the drug from its receptor sites, so that subsequent doses of the drug are unable to form the drug–receptor complexes which are required to produce an effect. Alternatively the drug may exert its response through the release of an endogenous mediator whose stores become rapidly depleted with consecutive doses of the drug.

There are several instances where the apparent tolerance to drugs cannot be explained in such simple terms and where other factors are evidently involved. A number of drugs acting on the central nervous system, particularly the group known as the narcotic analgesics, produce tolerance which is accompanied by physical dependence. This is a state in which an abrupt termination of the administration of the drug produces a series of unpleasant symptoms known as the abstinence syndrome. These symptoms are rapidly reversed after the readministration of the drug. A further manifestation of this problem involves psychogenic dependence in which the drug taker experiences an irreversible craving, or compulsion, to take the drug for pleasure or for the relief of discomfort.

Where more than one drug is being taken there is a possibility for a drug interaction to occur. Less commonly, drugs may interact with certain foodstuffs. These interactions are in the main, well documented. Their effects can range from minor toxicity to potential fatality. Such interactions may occur at the site of absorption where one agent may increase or decrease the rate or extent of absorption of the other. Alternatively drug interactions may affect the distribution metabolism or excretion of the interacting drugs. These types of interaction are known as pharmacokinetic drug interactions. A second type is the pharmacodynamic drug interaction where one drug can affect the response of another drug at its site of action.

The use of drugs in sport

Any discussion on drugs in sport should not be confined to the problem of drug misuse for performance enhancing purposes. Within a sporting context, a drug may have been taken for a variety of reasons, the more common of which are listed below:

1. Legitimate therapeutic purposes.
2. Performance continuation.
3. Recreational use.
4. Performance enhancement.

Inevitably, clear distinctions cannot always be made between these various uses. This may have important repercussions particularly when drugs are being taken at the time when the athlete is involved in competition.

LEGITIMATE THERAPEUTIC USE OF DRUGS

As with any member of the general public, a sportsman or woman is liable to suffer from a major or minor ailment that requires treatment with drugs. A typical example might involve a bacterial or fungal infection of a tissue necessitating the use of an antibiotic or antifungal agent. How many sportsmen have experienced athlete's foot? Apart from the slight risk of side effects due to the drug, it is difficult to perceive how such a drug would affect an athlete's performance. A less common, but more serious, medical condition would be epilepsy or diabetes. Under these circumstances it would be inconceivable for an athlete to consider participating in sport without regular treatment with drugs.

For many minor illnesses, from which we all suffer from time to time, such as coughs, colds, gastrointestinal upsets, hay fever, a visit to the doctor is unnecessary. As an alternative, many people will turn to self medication. There is a wide range of preparations available for the treatment of minor illnesses which are readily available for purchase from a pharmacy, without the need for a doctor's prescription. The drugs that such medicines contain are relatively less potent than those drugs available on prescription only. Nonetheless, it is important for the sportsman to appreciate that some of these preparations contain drugs which are included in the list of the IOC Medical Commission's banned substances. Examples of such drugs include the psychomotor stimulant, caffeine; the sympathomimetic amines, ephedrine, pseudoephedrine, phenylpropanolamine and phenylephrine; and the narcotic analgesic, codeine. Though the dose levels of these drugs within the medicines are low, the sophisticated methods used for the analysis of drugs are capable of easily detecting these drugs or their metabolites in urine samples. It is, therefore, unwise for a sportsman to use such remedies, especially since there are many alternative forms of treatment or medication which do not include banned substances. It is also in the athlete's interest, in the event of visiting a medical practitioner, that the nature of any drug treatment is discussed with the doctor to avoid the prescribing of banned drugs wherever possible.

In Britain, the Sports Council have produced a leaflet entitled *Proposed List of Medicines which may be taken by competing sportsmen*. This list, which contains both those medicines available only on prescription and those available for purchase from a pharmacy, is intended to help sportsmen avoid banned substances.

PERFORMANCE CONTINUATION

Sportsmen and women frequently experience injuries involving muscles, ligaments and tendons. Provided that the injury is not too serious, it is common for the sufferer to take palliative treatment in the form of analgesic drugs. This enables the athlete to continue to train and even compete during the period of recovery from the injury. The wisdom of such action is perhaps open to question but the use of analgesics under these circumstances is unlikely to be construed as conferring an unfair advantage over fellow competitors. Similarly, drug treatment to alleviate the symptoms of minor ailments, such as sore throats, colds and stomach upsets can be seen as simply allowing an athlete to continue performing during a temporary adverse situation.

RECREATIONAL USE

Alcohol is a drug which has become sociably acceptable by many cultures throughout the world. It is capable of producing profound pharmacological effects and, in common with all drugs, elicits both short-term and chronic side effects. Increasingly, the drugs of abuse or 'street drugs' are being taken for 'recreational' purposes. These may range from the relatively soft drugs, such as marijuana, to the hard, addictive drugs such as the narcotic analgesics related to heroin and morphine and the psychomotor stimulants such as cocaine.

Marijuana (cannabis) is a drug derived from the hemp plant and which is normally taken by inhalation in the form of a cigarette ('joint'), but can be taken orally. The precise mode of action of cannabis is not fully understood but the effects produced are principally euphoria and elation accompanied by a loss of perception of time and space. Conflicting opinions exist on the dangers associated with prolonged use of cannabis. There is evidence that short-term recall memory can be impaired and that permanent brain damage may be induced.

The narcotic analgesics are readily absorbed when taken orally, by injection or by inhalation. They are potent drugs whose effects are primarily on the central nervous system. They depress certain centres of the brain resulting in reduced powers of concentration, fear and anxiety. Prolonged pain, more so than acute pain, is reduced. Some centres of the brain, such as the vomiting centre and those associated with salivation, sweating and bronchial secretion, are initially stimulated, though become depressed on continued use of the drugs. The respiratory and cough centres are depressed. Respiration becomes slow, it deepens and may be periodic in nature. Death as a result of overdose of narcotic analgesics normally occurs through respiratory depression. Characteristic side effects of narcotic analgesics include constricted pupil size, dry mouth, heaviness of the limbs, skin itchiness, suppression of hunger and constipation.

The recent discovery of opiatic receptors within the brain has helped in the understanding of the mode of action of morphine, heroin and other related narcotic analgesics. They appear to be mimicking the effect of certain endogenous opiates, known as endorphins and encephalin.

Narcotic analgesics are renowned for their ability to cause tolerance and dependence in the regular user. Tolerance to the drugs occurs over a period of time and increasing dose levels are needed to produce the same pharmacological effect. Dependence on narcotic analgesics leads to physical withdrawal symptoms. Symptoms normally begin with sweating, yawning and running of the eyes and nose. These are followed by a period of restlessness which leads to insomnia, nausea, vomiting and diarrhoea. This is accompanied by dilation of the pupils, muscular cramp and a 'goose flesh' feeling of the skin. Relief from the physical withdrawal symptoms of narcotic analgesics can be achieved by the re-administration of these drugs, hence the difficulty that addicts experience in trying to terminate their dependence on narcotic analgesics.

Though taken for recreational purposes, the effects of these drugs may well be manifested in the field of sport. Some sporting events even take place in an environment where alcohol is freely available both to the spectator and the performer. In other instances recreational drugs may have been taken with no intent to alter performance but the repercussions for the drug taker or his fellow competitors could be significant, especially where aggressive instincts are altered. Perhaps the most widely used recreational drug is caffeine, which is present in many of the beverages that we consume daily. These include tea, coffee, colas and other soft drinks. At the levels at which caffeine is normally consumed its pharmacological effects are minimal. However, attempts have been made to use caffeine as a doping agent by taking supplements in the form of tablets or injections. This has necessitated the introduction into the doping control regulations of an upper limit for caffeine present in urine samples.

PERFORMANCE ENHANCING DRUGS

This particular area of drug use is potentially the most serious threat to the credibility of competitive sport and has become the subject of doping control regulations. It concerns the deliberate, illigitimate use of drugs in an attempt to gain an unfair advantage over fellow competitors.

It would be appropriate, at this point, to provide a definition of a performance enhancing drug. Unfortunately a precise definition is extremely difficult to formulate for a number of reasons.

1. A particular drug which may be considered performance enhancing in one sport may well be deleterious to performance in another sport. Drugs with a sedative action, such as alcohol and beta blockers, would be considered useful in events such as rifle shooting where a reduced heart rate and steady stance are important. However, these drugs would be counter productive, if not dangerous, in most other sports.
2. Should performance enhancing drugs be defined by the fact that they are 'synthetic' or 'unnatural' substances to the body? This type of definition would exclude testosterone and other naturally occurring hormones which are used for illicit purposes. 'Blood doping', the method by which runners store quantities of their own blood in a

frozen state and re-infuse it prior to competing, in an attempt to increase oxygen carrying capacity, would also be excluded by such a definition.
3. Should substances used in special diets, such as vitamin supplements be classed as performance enhancing drugs?
4. Perhaps the greatest difficulty in precisely defining performance enhancing drugs concerns the prescribing and use of drugs which can be perceived as possessing performance enhancing properties but which are used for legitimate therapeutic purposes. This problem is readily illustrated when considering athletes who suffer from asthma. One of the most important classes of drugs used for their treatment is the group of bronchodilators, many of which are sympathomimetics and therefore the subject of doping control. Since asthmatic attacks are frequently associated with stress, of which competitive exercise is an extreme case, then this obviously produces severe problems for the asthmatic if they are to avoid transgressing the dope control regulations. Selected bronchodilator sympathomimetics are allowed under dope control regulations.

Performance enhancing drugs whether or not they are taken for the deliberate purpose of gaining an unfair advantage in sport are subject to doping control regulations. Although individual sports federations may include their own minor amendments, it is the International Olympic Committee's list of banned substances which is generally accepted for doping control procedures.

For many years the IOC's Medical Commission classified the banned substances into five categories, according to their mode of action. These five categories were:

1. Psychomotor stimulant drugs.
2. Sympathomimetic amines.
3. Miscellaneous central nervous system stimulants.
4. Narcotic analgesics.
5. Anabolic steroids.

In response to changing trends in the use of drugs in sport, the IOC has recently revised its classification of doping agents and methods. The list which was revised in 1986 is shown in Table 1. These groups of drugs are considered in greater detail in subsequent chapters of this book.

For each of the groups of drugs the IOC lists examples of the drugs falling within that group. The lists of drugs are not comprehensive but

Table 1 International Olympic Committee list of doping classes and methods

---

I   Doping classes
    A. Stimulants
    B. Narcotic analgesics
    C. Anabolic steroids
    D. Beta blockers
    E. Diuretics

II Doping methods
    A. Blood doping
    B. Pharmacological, chemical and physical manipulation

III Classes of drugs subject to certain restrictions
    A. Alcohol
    B. Local anaesthetics
    C. Corticosteroids

---

include the rider 'and related compounds'. The principle reason for this is to ensure that every new drug which is introduced onto the market and which belongs to one of the groups of banned drugs is automatically included within the list. This avoids the need for a continual update of the lists and prevents an athlete from claiming that the latest drug which they have been taking is not included on the list of banned substances. The drugs are listed under their generic name, which identifies the particular chemical substance(s) the drug contains. However, the same drug may be manufactured and sold by several different drug companies throughout the world and each company will use their own commercial name to describe that drug; for example, the analgesic paracetamol (generic name) can be bought under the commercial names 'Hedex' or 'Panadol'.

The situation is further complicated where, as frequently occurs, a drug is combined with other drugs within a medication. This commonly occurs with sympathomimetics combined with other substances in cough remedies, though there are many other examples involving banned drugs. Paracetamol is available in medicines such as 'Syndol' and 'Parahypon' though in these preparations it is combined with caffeine and codeine, two drugs which are subject to doping control regulations.

It is, therefore, important that a competitor should carefully scrutinize the label on any medication which is being taken to ensure that a banned substance is not included in the medicine. Should there be any doubt, then the competitor should seek expert advice.

The mere presence of one of the banned drugs, or their major metabolites, in a urine sample taken at a sporting event would constitute an offence. In the case of caffeine, a common constituent of beverages, and testosterone, a naturally occurring hormone, a quantitative analysis of the urine is required. This will determine whether the drug is present in the urine in quantities significantly greater than those 'normally' found in urine.

It would be easy to say that athletes should avoid taking drugs, for any reason, particularly at a time of competition. It has been shown, however, that there are many circumstances where drug taking is advisable if not imperative for the general health and well-being of the athlete. Therefore it would be prudent for athletes to consider carefully the specific need for taking drugs and the full implications of their action.

The rationale for drug misuse in sport

There may be many reasons to prompt a sportsman to misuse drugs. In the case of the performance enhancing drugs, the type of drug selected will depend upon the drug's pharmacological action and the sport in which the athlete is competing. Some of the more obvious correlations are presented below. However, such a rational approach by sportsmen is not always evident because of the multivariant factors which lead the competitor to embark on performance enhancing drug-taking.

STIMULANT DRUGS

This group of drugs includes psychomotor stimulants, sympathomimetics and miscellaneous CNS stimulants which have a wide profile of pharmacological activity. They may produce alertness, wakefulness and an increase in the ability to concentrate. In addition, they may improve the faculty to exercise strenuously or produce a decreased sensitivity to pain. These effects are potentially of benefit to a wide variety of sports involving sustained physical and mental activity. However, there is little scientific evidence in the literature to suggest that these drugs improve performance.

Detrimentally, these drugs may make the athlete more aggressive and hostile to fellow competitors resulting in increased brutality in sports involving physical contact. Toxic side effects of these drugs include a tendency to habituation, rebound effects on withdrawal and the possibility of interaction with other drugs. The ability of some of these drugs to push back the natural limits of fatigue has lead to a number of cases of death through exhaustion and heat stroke.

NARCOTIC ANALGESICS

This group of powerful painkilling drugs enables athletes to exert themselves beyond their normal pain threshold. This, in itself, may pose a health hazard to a competitor who may be tempted to compete despite an existing serious injury which could result in more permanent physical damage to a tissue.

As these drugs have strong addictive properties, they are tightly controlled by legislation in most countries. An exception to this is the drug codeine, which is widely available in a variety of medicines, for example, analgesics, cough mixtures and cold remedies. These preparations can be bought over the counter in a pharmacy. The levels of codeine present in these medicines are too low to induce the serious adverse effects associated with the narcotic analgesics. This does, however, pose a problem for drug testing, since codeine is metabolized along a similar pathway to morphine. Differences in attitude exist between sports federations as to whether codeine should be prohibited as a doping substance. The IOC certainly includes codeine in its list of banned drugs.

ANABOLIC STEROIDS

This group of drugs is responsible for the most widespread abuse of drugs in sport. They are taken in extremely large doses by some athletes who are involved in weightlifting, throwing and many other sports involving strength. The pretext for using these drugs is to increase muscle development, though, apart from females and prepubital males, there is no strong evidence to show that these steroids exert a direct growth promoting effect on muscles.

The side effects associated with these drugs are extremely serious, particularly the consequences of their long-term use. This will be discussed in greater detail in Chapter 2. It is in the two groups of individuals who are most likely to derive the dubious benefit of muscular development that the greatest risk of toxic side effects occurs. Females will undergo masculinization resulting in hair growth on the face and body, irreversible voice changes, and serious disturbances to the menstrual cycle. Prepubital males may experience stunting of growth among other effects.

Unfortunately the reputation of anabolic steroids as performance enhancing drugs has achieved a considerable level of notoriety among certain athletes, whilst the adverse effects of these drugs, being of a more long-term nature, have been conveniently ignored. What is required is an extensive programme of education to warn athletes of the hazardous consequences of the use of anabolic steroids in a non-therapeutic manner.

BETA BLOCKERS AND OTHER DRUGS WITH A SEDATIVE ACTION

Several groups of drugs with widely differing modes of action are used in sports where physical effort is not paramount but where a calming effect is required, for example archery or shooting events.

Alcohol, in small amounts, may have a sedative effect but irregular consumption can lead to fluctuating blood alcohol levels. Alcohol is not a prohibited substance but certain international federations may require competitors to undergo breath or blood alcohol level determinations. Tranquillizers, particularly the benzodiazepines, are widely prescribed and consequently are relatively easy to obtain by sportsmen. It is fair to say that this particular group of drugs has a very low incidence of serious side effects. This group of drugs is not, at present, prohibited.

Beta blockers present a very interesting group of drugs. Their primary therapeutic use is in diseases of the cardiovascular system. Part of their mode of action is to reduce heart rate and cardiac output. This can be seen to have a beneficial performance-enhancing effect not only in shooting events but also for sports such as motor racing and ski jumping. One of the side effects of beta blockers is a tendency to induce sedation, which again can be turned to advantage in sports where a calming effect is desirable. Inevitably, the other common side effects of beta blockers such as sleep disturbances and cold hands militates against their use in sport. In view of the wide range of alternative drugs available for therapeutic control of disease states for which beta blockers are prescribed, the IOC has included beta blockers in its list of banned substances.

DIURETICS

The pharmacological effect of diuretics involves the elimination of fluid from the body and their use is indicated in a number of disease states. There are two main reasons why diuretics are sometimes misused by competitors. Firstly, they may be taken to effect a rapid reduction in weight, obviously a potential advantage in sports such as boxing or weightlifting where weight categories are involved. Secondly, diuretics are used to increase urine excretion at times when a competitor is liable to undergo a drug detection test. The resultant increase in urine volume will serve to dilute the doping agent, or its metabolites, within the urine. In view of the sophistication of drug detection techniques, this method of subterfuge is unlikely to be effective.

BLOOD DOPING

Blood doping does not involve the administration of drugs. Red blood cells or blood products containing red blood cells are administered intravenously in an attempt to gain unfair advantage in competition by increasing the blood's oxygen carrying capacity. The blood so used may have been drawn previously from the same individual or from a different donor. Apart from contravening the ethics of sport and medicine, this procedure carries tremendous risk to the individual recipient. Use of the competitor's own blood can overload the cardiovascular circulation and induce metabolic shock. These adverse effects are compounded if blood from a second individual is used, where an allergic reaction may develop or a mismatch in blood typing can lead to a potentially fatal haemolytic reaction with kidney failure. Increasingly, the recipient risks contracting infectious diseases such as AIDS or viral hepatitis.

LOCAL ANAESTHETICS

Local anaesthetics, with the exception of cocaine, are not banned substances provided their use is medically justified and their route of administration is either locally applied or by intra-articular injection. Where appropriate, details of the diagnosis, dose and route of administration of the local anaesthetic must be submitted, in writing, to the IOC Medical Commission or Sports Federation.

CORTICOSTEROIDS

Corticosteroids are naturally occurring or synthetically produced drugs which are related to the adrenocorticosteroid hormones released from the adrenal cortex. They should not be confused with anabolic steroids. Therapeutically they are used as analgesic and anti-inflammatory drugs. Corticosteroids produce several serious toxic effects if their use is prolonged or under inadequate medical control. These adverse effects are less likely to occur if the drugs are restricted to topical adminis-tration.

Consequently, the IOC has banned the use of corticosteroids except in topical preparations for ear, eye or skin conditions, for inhalation therapy in asthma and allergic rhinitis or for local or intra-articular injection. Where local or intra-articular injection is prescribed the team doctor must give written notification to the IOC Medical Commission.

The control of drug misuse in sport

The misuse of drugs in sport is condemned by most individuals involved in sport and most certainly by the IOC and other bodies concerned with sport administration. It is not sufficient merely to express condemnation of drug misuse, it is necessary to take steps to prevent such abuse and to sanction those who are found to have illicitly used drugs in sport. To this end the IOC and Sports Federations now require competitors to undergo simple testing procedures to establish whether an individual has been involved in illicit drug taking. These tests are normally carried out on a random sampling procedure at major sporting events, though increasingly, administrating bodies are introducing out-of-season random drug testing programmes. The lists of banned substances have already been referred to in this chapter. It is important to note that those lists only include drugs for which an effective method of detection is available, since it would be folly to ban a substance for which no proof of it having been taken can be presented in evidence. There is no detection method, at present, for blood doping.

The responsibility for organizing drugs testing lies with the governing bodies of individual sports. In Britain, the national organization of drug testing is undertaken by the Sports Council who require national governing bodies to submit evidence of effective doping control regulations as a condition of the grant and services they receive from the

Sports Council. The procedures for processing samples for analysis is normally placed with an accredited drug testing centre. Accreditation is dependent upon adequate facilities being available at the centre, both in terms of their range and capability of the analytical equipment and also the capacity of the centre for testing the numbers of samples required for a comprehensive control system. For major sporting events it is sometimes necessary to assemble a drug testing centre specifically for that event.

PROCEDURES FOR DRUG TESTING IN SPORT

Sample collection

The testing for drugs requires the athlete to provide a sample of urine for analysis. The selection procedures for sample collection are normally on a random basis. Where the testing is carried out at a sporting event many governing bodies specify that the winner in each event plus a number of other competitors, selected at random, will be tested. Out-of-season testing is also made on a random basis and normally requires collection by a sampling officer at a training session.

Athletes selected for testing, at a competitive event, are normally notified by an official at the event. They are asked to sign a form to acknowledge that they have been notified and that they agree to the test. Sample collection is made at a control station. Refusal to undergo drug testing, or failure to attend at the control station, is deemed an admission of guilt and the athlete is considered to have provided a positive urine test. The procedures normally adopted for a positive result would then ensue. However, there would be no possibility for a second confirmatory analysis to be carried out. The athlete may be accompanied by a team manager or other official at the Control Station. The urine sample is collected under supervision. A sufficient volume of urine is taken to provide a sample for the primary test and a further sample for a second test should the first test prove positive. Problems may be encountered in producing a sufficient volume of urine particularly when an athlete is dehydrated after competing; however, drinks are supplied and sufficient time is allowed for the sample to be taken. The length of time sometimes involved between completion of an event and the provision of a urine sample at the Control Station has led to problems in the past with athletes substituting 'clean' urine samples in place of their own. Particular vigilance is therefore required by the supervising staff at this stage in the procedure. The athlete is allowed to check that the sample has been correctly marked and sealed, then normally signs a form indicating his satisfaction with the collection procedure.

Sample analysis

Samples collected at the Control Station are taken under close supervision to the drug testing centre for analysis. The procedures for analysis should be completed as soon as possible after arrival at the laboratory, again observing the strictest level of security.

The techniques used for the analysis of drugs first involve the extraction of the drugs into appropriate solvents. Most drugs are detected using chromatographic methods, principally gas–liquid chromatography (GLC) and high performance liquid chromatography (HPLC). These methods involve the absorption of the chemical constituents of the sample onto a stationary phase of the apparatus. The moving phase of the system, a gas or liquid, then displaces these chemicals at different times, under different physical conditions. The chemicals leaving the apparatus are monitored with a detection instrument and the peaks on the chart are compared with those of known standard drugs. This allows for the presumptive identification of the compound. Both the drug taken and, where appropriate, its metabolites, can be detected in this manner. It has been known for athletes to take substances which are not, in themselves, banned but whose purpose is to disguise an illegal drug present in the urine sample. This is achieved when the two compounds produce similar peaks following chromatography. There are few cases where this subterfuge applies but to double check, gas chromatography is accompanied by a second technique known as mass spectrometry. Using this double method the compounds are isolated by gas chromatography and then, using mass spectrometry, the compounds are bombarded with a beam of electrons resulting in ionization of the molecules which can then be recorded on a mass spectrum. This allows a true characterization of the compound.

For routine screening, the drug testing laboratories use the more economical GLC, thin layer chromatography (TLC) and HPLC methods and reserve the more complex and expensive method of gas chromatography/mass spectrometry for situations where interference is a problem or where confirmation of a suspect sample is required. The results of gas chromatography/mass spectometry are vital as evidence in any court proceedings resulting from drug testing.

Immunoassay is another technique which is more specific than GLC or TLC. This method involves the production of antisera which are designed to react with specific compounds present in urine as a result of drug taking. The greater the concentration of compound present in the urine, the less free antiserum will remain. Since the antisera are labelled with radioisotopes or enzymes they can be easily detected. Therefore, the levels of drug or metabolites in the urine can be indirectly measured using this technique.

Results of analysis

In the event of a negative result, where no banned substances are found in the urine, a report is sent to the governing body who requested the test. The urine samples are then destroyed.

A positive result will be reported to the governing body of the sport, who will, in turn, notify the athlete. Subsequent events may vary but in general the following procedures are adopted. The athlete is suspended from competing in events organized by the governing body in question pending further investigations. Initially the athlete will be questioned as to why the drug was present in the urine sample. The athlete also has the right to a repeat analysis of the second urine sample taken at the time of the event. The athlete and a representative are entitled to observe this repeat analysis.

Having weighed all the evidence the governing body will take a decision which may include suspension from competition for a period of time or even a lifetime ban. Medals may be withdrawn. The athlete will always have the right to appeal against a decision, to an authorized body. The severity of the penalty imposed upon an athlete will of course depend on the perceived degree of gravity or intent. Any sportsman found guilty and subsequently suspended should be continuously re-checked during the period of suspension if he or she intends to return to competitive sport. The IOC have recommended guidelines for sanctions to be applied in positive cases which differentiate between 'deliberate' and 'inadvertant' doping.

Increasing support is being given for the imposition of life bans at international level as an effective way of dealing with drug abuse within sport. One way of helping to implement such a proposal would be to persuade the IOC and the international sports federations to draw up stricter eligibility rules; this would prevent banned athletes from competing at high levels of competition.

The guilt associated with the misuse of drugs in sport does not always lie entirely with the athlete. Complicity by medical doctors, coaches and other persons associated with the individual or team involved in drug misuse is common. It is equally, if not more, important that penalties should be directed towards such persons, particularly where their influence extends to younger athletes. Sanctions against coaches, doctors, etc. who have been shown to be involved in illegal drug supply to athletes should certainly include withdrawal of their official recognition from sport. Where applicable, action might also be taken under their own professional code of conduct.

Avoiding detection

Recent reports suggest that athletes and their medical advisers are showing increasing ingenuity in their attempts to avoid detection during random drug testing. One method adopted is to use probenecid to disguise the fact that anabolic steroids are being taken. Probenecid is a drug used in the prophylactic treatment of gout. An alternative therapeutic use for probenecid is in combination with some antibodies to increase their plasma concentrations and prolong their antibacterial effects. Probenecid achieves this effect by blocking the excretion of the antibiotics through the renal tubules in the kidneys.

Certain competitors are using probenecid to inhibit the excretion of anabolic steroids and their metabolites. Urine levels of the steroids are thereby reduced thus decreasing the chances of detection when urine is screened. The drug is therefore taken at times when random drug testing is likely to occur. This has led to the inclusion of probenecid as a banned substance.

Another method being used by some athletes in an attempt to avoid detection is to take human chorionic gonadotrophin. This substance is derived from the urine of pregnant women and is used clinically to treat infertility. The male hormone testosterone, occurs naturally in the body but is classed as a banned substance when taken for purposes of increasing muscle mass. Human chorionic gonadotrophin, which is on the banned list, is taken to stimulate the body's production of testosterone.

A further preparation, occasionally used, is human growth hormone. This hormone is used clinically to treat dwarfism in children and has a stimulating effect on growth in all tissues. Human growth hormone is very expensive and difficult to obtain. This can lead to a further sinister aspect associated with drug abuse in sport, that of obtaining supplies by theft.

Anabolic steroids probably present the greatest threat to the future credibility of spectator sport. They are the most widely used, and in the long term the most toxic, of the substances abused. At present, anabolic steroids are only available on a doctor's prescription, and their use in Britain, is controlled by the Medicines Act. This act is mainly concerned with consumer protection. If these drugs were to be controlled under the Misuse of Drugs Act then there would be greater powers to control their illegal use. Additionally, it would become possible to prosecute those found trafficing in anabolic steroids. This transfer of legal control would classify anabolic steroids alongside drugs such as heroin and cocaine. Therefore the use of anabolic steroids by persons who had not obtained them through a doctor's prescription would constitute a criminal act.

A consequence of this tighter legislative control of anabolic steroids would be that the present system for testing these drugs, in Britain, would be unacceptable in law. This may well prompt the setting up of an independent drug testing agency which would probably be under direct governmental control. The involvement of such an independent agency would certainly curtail the currently rumoured practice of protecting selected sports stars against ill-timed random drug testing. Such rumours have implicated officials and sponsors as having succumbed to blackmail from athletes who threaten to pull out of events where a risk of their being drug-tested exists.

Attitudes towards drugs in sport

There are many reasons why an athlete may take a drug, other than for legitimate therapeutic purposes. Previous experiences, at school or college, may prompt further experimentation with drugs within a sporting context. This approach may easily be fuelled by an athlete reading about drugs and their effects in popular magazines or even in serious scientific journals. Unfortunately, too many people involved in sport, at all levels, are prepared to speculate through television, newspapers or other media on the problem of drug abuse in sport. Too often these unsubstantiated reports lead to accusations and counter-accusations between those involved in the practice and administration of sport. Such activities do little to enhance the reputation of sport and inevitably lead to confusion in the minds of the majority of sportsmen and women who do not take 'performance enhancing' drugs. This uncertainty presents the greatest danger to those younger athletes who either become disenchanted with their chosen sport or are misled into believing that drug taking has become a necessary part of the route to sporting success. Other athletes may experience pressure from peer groups, particularly fellow athletes from their own or other sports. This pressure may result from a desire to conform with the 'in-crowd'. Alternatively, it may be a fear of competing, on unequal terms, with athletes who are suspected of taking drugs.

A different type of psychological pressure may be involved in another group of athletes. For these athletes, drug taking may be the last resort for the improvement of performance, having reached their apparent limit of capability by conventional methods of training.

The motivating factors for drug misuse do not necessarily lie in the hands of the athlete. It is an unfortunate fact that certain athletes are coerced into taking drugs by someone in authority. This person may be their coach, trainer or team doctor. The directive may even have originated from a country's governing body. Such pressures are obviously extremely difficult to resist, particularly where team selection is at stake. Many studies have been carried out, using questionnaires, to ascertain attitudes towards drugs in sport. From these studies, the majority of athletes, coaches, medical practitioners and others involved in sport do not favour the use of performance enhancing drugs. However, these results may reflect the respondent's ethical and moral attitudes to the problem but in practice, the pressures of competition may compel them to take a more pragmatic approach to drug taking. This denial of drug taking is a common feature among alcohol and drug abusers and further hinders any attempt at tackling the problem. Potentially more damaging is the type of athlete who openly admits to taking drugs and by so doing provides a model for younger, more impressionable athletes to follow.

The blame for taking drugs does not of course always lie entirely with the athlete. There is often a body of so-called 'enablers' such as friends, family, coaches, etc. who either actively encourage the athlete to participate in drug taking or vehemently shield the user from the need to deal with the problem. The reasons for this attitute are not always clear but in most cases involve self interest. Conversely, those closely associated with the athlete may be unaware of their drug abusing habits. This may, to a large extent, be due to a lack of knowledge and understanding of the drugs used and of their pharmacological effects.

It is clear that the majority of those involved in sport, both administrators and participants, are against the misuse of drugs in sport. It is equally clear that there is too little understanding of both the motivating factors that lead an athlete to take drugs and also the effects that those drugs can induce. It is vital that a wider knowledge, of drugs and their adverse effects, is achieved so that the current problem of drug abuse in sport can be contained and that future generations can be educated and persuaded against such misuse.

1 Sympathomimetic amines and their antagonists

D. J. ARMSTRONG

1.1 Summary

The sympathetic nervous system controls many aspects of bodily function including cardiac function, blood pressure, airway diameter and the somatic manifestations of anxiety. Consequently, drugs which either mimic or block the sympathetic nervous system have considerable potential for abuse. The commonest therapeutic uses of sympathomimetic drugs are in the treatment of asthma and coughs and colds. The possible stimulation of both the cardiovascular system and the central nervous system by some drugs in this class has led to their being banned by the IOC. Beta-adrenoceptor blocking drugs (antagonists) are widely used to treat high blood pressure and angina pectoris. It is important that patients who are receiving these drugs understand the effects they have upon performance and tolerance of exercise. Beta blockers reduce the symptoms of anxiety which are mediated by the sympathetic nervous system, e.g. muscle tremor. The potential for abuse exists in those activities in which fine motor control is more important than oxygen utilization, e.g. snooker, shooting and archery. Alpha-adrenoceptor antagonists, although commonly prescribed for the treatment of hypertension, are not the subject of abuse in sport.

Sympathomimetic amines are drugs which mimic the effects of noradrenaline and adrenaline which in turn are the naturally occurring (endogenous) agonists of the sympathetic nervous system (SNS). Antagonists are drugs which block the effects of the agonists.

1.2 Anatomy and physiology of the autonomic nervous system (ANS)

The autonomic nervous system (ANS) is divided into the parasympathetic and sympathetic branches. The parasympathetic nervous system is that branch of the ANS which is responsible for controlling many bodily functions under normal resting conditions. The sympathetic nervous system (SNS) is that branch of the ANS which prepares the body for what is often referred to as the fight/flight or fright response, i.e. it increases cardiac activity, dilates the airways, increases blood sugar concentrations but slows down digestion and the passage of food through the gastrointestinal tract.

The SNS consists of parts of the brainstem and the spinal cord, certain nerves arising from the spinal cord and the adrenal glands. Because the sympathetic nerves arise principally from the thoracic and lumbar regions of the spinal cord, this branch of the ANS is referred to as the thoracolumbar division of the ANS. The nerves of the parasympathetic nervous system (PNS) arise from the brainstem and the sacral region of the spinal cord and is referred to, therefore, as the craniosacral division of the ANS.

The sympathetic nerves do not go directly from the spinal cord to the target glands or effectors, e.g. the heart and lungs, etc. Instead they make synapses with a second order of neurones in structures known as ganglia, which lie adjacent to the spinal cord and which form the paravertebral chain. Nerves between the spinal cord and the ganglia are pre-ganglionic nerves and those between ganglia and the effectors are post-ganglionic. The junctions between neurones and between neurones and effectors are synapses. The transmitter released by the pre-ganglionic nerve fibres is acetylcholine, consideration of which is beyond the scope of this chapter. The neurotransmitter released by the

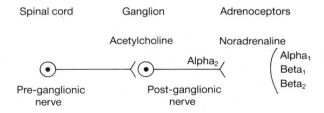

Figure 1.1 The distribution of pre- and post-synaptic adrenoceptors.

Table 1.1 The effects of the sympathetic nervous system

Effector	Receptor	Response
Heart		
S-A node	Beta$_1$	↑ Heart rate
Ventricles	Beta$_1$	↑ Force of contraction
Lungs		
Bronchial muscle	Alpha$_1$	Contraction
Bronchial muscle	Beta$_2$	Relaxation
Blood vessels		
Coronary	Alpha$_1$	Constriction
	Beta$_2$	Dilatation
Skeletal muscle	Alpha$_1$	Constriction
	Beta$_2$	Dilatation
Skin	Alpha$_1$	Constriction
Renal	Alpha$_1$	Constriction
GIT		
Motility	Beta$_1$	↓ Contraction
Liver	Beta$_2$	Glycogenolysis
Pancreas	Alpha$_1$	↓ Insulin
	Beta$_2$	↑ Insulin
Adipose tissue	Beta$_2$	Lipolysis
Eye		
Radial muscle of iris	Alpha$_1$	Contraction (mydriasis)
Ciliary muscle	Beta$_2$	Relaxation for distant vision

post-ganglionic nerves of the SNS is noradrenaline (Figure 1.1). The effects of noradrenaline are supplemented by adrenaline which is released from the chromaffin cells in the medullae of the adrenal glands.

Noradrenaline and adrenaline exert different effects on the body because they affect different receptors on cells in tissues and organs (Table 1.1).

The classification of adrenoceptors was first defined by Alhquist in

1948. Adrenoceptors are defined on the basis of those drugs that stimulate them, i.e. agonists, and those drugs that block or antagonize them, i.e. antagonists. Alpha receptors are those that demonstrate the following sensitivity to agonists: adrenaline > noradrenaline ≫ isoprenaline (a synthetic sympathomimetic drug). Beta receptors demonstrate a different sensitivity: isoprenaline > adrenaline > noradrenaline.

Classification of adrenoceptors has been extended to two sub-types of both alpha and beta adrenoceptors based upon sensitivity to selective agonists:

Receptor	Location	Agonist
Alpha$_1$	Post-synaptic alpha receptors	Phenylephrine
Alpha$_2$	Pre-synaptic alpha receptors	Clonidine
Beta$_1$	Post-synaptic beta receptors	Noradrenaline
Beta$_2$	Post-synaptic beta receptors	Salbutamol

The adrenoceptors subserve different functions, depending upon their location, e.g. stimulation of alpha$_1$ receptors causes vasoconstriction; alpha$_2$ receptors inhibit the release of noradrenaline from postganglionic sympathetic nerves; beta$_1$ receptors increase the rate and force of contraction of heart muscle; stimulation of beta$_2$ receptors causes bronchodilatation.

1.3 Adrenergic agonists

1.3.1 ENDOGENOUS AGONISTS

Adrenaline (epinephrine) is the hormone released from the adrenal medullae during stress. It stimulates alpha$_1$, alpha$_2$, beta$_1$ and beta$_2$ receptors. Beta$_1$-receptor stimulation increases heart rate, myocardial contractility and hence increases cardiac output. Stimulation of alpha$_1$ receptors causes vasoconstriction and raises systolic arterial blood pressure. Stimulation of beta$_2$ receptors in blood vessels in skeletal muscle causes vasodilation and may decrease peripheral resistance and hence cause a fall in diastolic blood pressure. Neurogenic vasodilatation during exercise will be supplemented by humoral vasodilatation in the exercising muscles. The magnitude of this response is directly related to the exercising muscle mass. Adrenaline also increases respiratory rate, tidal volume and hence minute ventilation. It is an effective, rapidly acting bronchodilator (15 min) through stimulation of beta$_2$ receptors.

The duration of action is between 60 and 90 minutes after either subcutaneous injection or inhalation from a pressurized aerosol. Stimulation of alpha$_1$ receptors causes vasoconstriction and reduces the inflammation and oedema in the bronchial lining of the asthmatic. These two mechanisms make adrenaline an effective prophylactic therapy for exercise-induced asthma and the drug of choice for the emergency treatment of exercise-induced anaphylaxis (Eisenstadt *et al.*. 1984). However, because of its cardiovascular effects it is banned by the IOC.

Noradrenaline (norepinephrine) is the neurotransmitter at sympathetic nerve endings. It has similar effects to adrenaline on beta$_1$ receptors in the heart. However, it is a less potent agonist of alpha receptors and has little effect on beta$_2$ receptors. It is contraindicated for the treatment of asthma. It increases peripheral vascular resistance, systolic and diastolic arterial blood pressures and cardiac output. It is banned by the IOC although it is rarely used therapeutically.

1.3.2 SYMPATHOMIMETIC AMINES

These are manufactured drugs which mimic the actions of the sympathetic nervous system, primarily through stimulating one or more adrenoceptors. Examples include ephedrine and isoprenaline.

Unlike adrenaline and isoprenaline, ephedrine is active orally. It has high bioavailability and ten times the duration of action of adrenaline. It is less likely to cause tachycardia but causes greater CNS stimulation than adrenaline. Ephedrine is only a weak bronchodilator. Its primary mode of action is the release of stored catecholamines, i.e. adrenaline and noradrenaline. It is commonly used as a topical nasal decongestant and is included in numerous cough and cold remedies but is rarely used to treat asthma. It is banned by the IOC because of its cardiac stimulant and amphetamine-like CNS stimulant activity.

Isoprenaline is a potent beta-receptor agonist that has little effect upon alpha receptors. When applied as an aerosol, it is a potent bronchodilator. Indeed, it was the original beta agonist to be used as a topical bronchodilator. It also serves as the best example of the problems inherent in the use of a non-selective beta agonist. Although stimulation of beta$_2$ receptors causes bronchodilatation, simultaneous stimulation of beta$_1$ receptors increases heart rate to potentially dangerous levels. Since an asthmatic attack causes great anxiety, heart rate will already be elevated by increased sympathetic nervous system activity and the circumstances are ideal for the induction of cardiac arrhythmia. Indeed, following the introduction of isoprenaline in the 1960s there was a significant increase in the incidence of fatal cardiac arrhythmias in those asthmatics treated with inhaled isoprenaline. Whether this was due to incorrect use/abuse of the drug or to the inherent problems of a non-selective beta agonist has been the subject of much inconclusive debate. Like adrenaline and ephedrine, the use of isoprenaline in competition is banned by the IOC.

There are many other examples of sympathomimetic amines. Those relevant to sport are discussed below.

Sympathomimetic amines have many therapeutic indications including: asthma; cough and cold remedies; anaphylactic shock; cardiogenic shock; paroxysmal atrial tachycardia; drug overdoses which cause hypotension; local anaesthetic preparations; topical nasal decongestants (Katzung, 1987). Perhaps the most important therapeutic use of these drugs and that which has greatest potential for abuse in sport, is the treatment of asthma.

Asthma and its treatment

Asthma is a disease which is characterized by widespread narrowing of the peripheral airways which in the early stages can be paroxysmal and reversible. There are numerous causes of asthma, e.g. allergy, drugs, occupational pollution, emotion, stress, infection. Exercise can also induce an asthmatic attack in susceptible individuals. The treatment of exercise-induced asthma will be considered at the end of this section. Despite the multiplicity of causes, asthma is normally classified into extrinsic and intrinsic.

Extrinsic asthma is the commonest type of asthma in children. There is often a family history of allergic conditions, e.g. eczema, hay fever and asthma itself. The patient will commonly exhibit a positive skin prick test although not in all cases. Those individuals who are positive are termed atopic but not all atopic individuals are asthmatics. Approximately 2–5% of the population have asthma whilst some 30% of the population are atopic. The commonest allergens are either grass or tree pollens and the droppings of the house dust mite (*Dermatophagoides pteronyssinus*). This is the best understood form of asthma. Inhaled or ingested allergens (reaginic antigens) bind to IgE antibodies which are on the surface of mast cells. Mast cells have been identified in the bronchial lumen, epithelium and submucosa. The antigen–antibody reaction stimulates the release from mast cells both of preformed mediators which were contained in granules (e.g. histamine) and membrane-derived mediators (e.g. leukotrienes, LTC_4, LTD_4, LTE_4 and platelet activating factor (PAF)). In the acute phase, this causes bronchoconstriction and an asthma attack. In severe chronic asthma, this can cause hypersensitivity of airway smooth muscle, secretion of tenacious mucus, inflammation and oedema of the bronchial wall (Clark, 1983).

In intrinsic asthma the patient has asthma but does not exhibit a positive skin prick test. Onset of symptoms tends to be later in life (4th and 5th decades) and there is no family history of atopy. The levels of IgE are not elevated and the cause of asthma is not well understood. Intrinsic asthma is generally more refractory to treatment than extrinsic asthma.

The treatment of asthma falls into 2 categories – prophylactic (preventative) and bronchodilator (relief of symptoms).

Prophylactic treatment of asthma

1. Avoidance of allergens or 'trigger factors'. If the asthmatic can be shown to be hypersensitive to either an inhaled or an ingested allergen then exposure should be reduced to an absolute minimum. This will help to reduce the frequency of the attacks.

2. Sodium cromoglycate (SCG). This is one of the safest of drugs and forms the first line of treatment of allergic asthma. It is more effective in children than adults. Administration is by inhalation of dry powder, by aerosol or nebuliser. The only common side-effect is generation of a cough by inhalation of the dry powder. This can be circumvented by either aerosol, if the patient can use one correctly, or by prior administration of a $beta_2$ agonist. SCG stabilizes the membrane of mast cells and prevents the release of the mediators of bronchoconstriction. It must be emphasized to the patient that this prevents bronchoconstriction but does not cause bronchodilatation of constricted airways. Consequently, it will not relieve the symptoms of an attack. They should use the drug continually, not just when symptoms are present. If this is not explained to the patient then they may dismiss the drug as being ineffective. However, it is ineffective in more than 90% of intrinsic asthmatics. Most of these patients will eventually require long-term steroid therapy, either inhaled or oral. SCG has no effect on the cardiovascular system and is of no ergogenic value. Its use is permitted by the IOC.

3. Steroids. Glucocorticoids are an essential component of the treatment of asthma in many individuals although they are considered to be the last line of therapy for severe asthmatics who do not respond to the other anti-asthma drugs. In emergencies they can be life saving. Although their value is unquestioned, their mode of action is largely unknown. They decrease the swelling and oedema of the inflamed bronchial mucosa, mucus secretion and airway hypersensitivity whilst increasing the sensitivity to beta$_2$ agonists. Steroids may be administered orally, by injection or by inhalation. Oral and intravenous steroids produce many unwanted side effects. Inhaled steroids (betamethasone, beclamethasone and budesonide) can be used to replace oral steroids in many asthmatics and are without systemic side effects in therapeutic doses. They are, therefore, the formulation of choice for administration of steroids. Inhaled/topical steroids are unlikely to have any ergogenic effects and are permitted by the IOC. The glucocorticoid group of steroid hormones have different effects from those of the anabolic steroids which are discussed in Chapter 2.

Bronchodilator therapy

There are three groups of drugs which are used to relax the constricted airways of the asthmatic during an attack. These drugs are therefore used to treat the symptoms rather than to prevent an attack from occurring.

1. Selective beta$_2$ agonists. The first beta agonist to be used in the treatment of asthma was isoprenaline. The problems with isoprenaline prompted the development of a new generation of selective beta$_2$ agonists for use as bronchodilators. These are listed in Table 1.2. Only the first three are permitted under IOC regulations (Table 1.3).

   All the selective beta$_2$ agonists are potent bronchodilators. There are only minor differences between the pharmacological profiles of these drugs but salbutamol is the yardstick against which other beta$_2$ agonists are assessed. There are many formulations of salbutamol and terbutaline including tablets, slow-release tablets, elixirs, aerosols and dry powders, solutions for injection and inhalation from a nebuliser. At the time of publication, there were fewer formulations of other beta$_2$ agonists although this is likely to change. All but

Table 1.2 Selective beta$_2$-adrenoceptor agonists

Salbutamol (Ventolin) (albuterol, USA)
Terbutaline (Bricanyl) (brethine, USA)
Rimiterol (Pulmadil)
Fenoterol (Berotec)
Pirbuterol (Exirel)

Table 1.3 Those sympathomimetics which may and may not be used under IOC regulations

Banned	Permitted*
Adrenaline	Salbutamol
Noradrenaline	Terbutaline
Ephedrine	Rimiterol
Isoprenaline	Orciprenaline
Fenoterol	Bitolterol

* Subject to written notification.

rimiterol and fenoterol are active after oral administration (Clark and Cochrane, 1984).

Tremor is the only common side effect after aerosol administration which is therefore the route of choice. The side effects after oral administration include: fine tremor (usually of the hands), nervous tension and headache. Tachycardia, peripheral vasodilatation and hypokalaemia may occur after oral dosing but are commoner after intravenous injection. Tachycardia is most uncommon after aerosol inhalation. Because of the greater speed of onset and the reduced incidence of side effects, aerosol administration is preferable to oral dosing. The duration of action after aerosol administration is approximately 6 hours for fenoterol, salbutamol and terbutaline but slightly less for rimiterol.

Selective beta$_2$ agonists are contraindicated in the presence of hyperthyroidism, hypertension and ischaemic heart disease. Intravenous administration is contraindicated by diabetes mellitus.

The IOC (1988) permits the use of salbutamol, terbutaline,

orciprenaline, bitolterol and rimiterol (subject to written notification) but not of fenoterol, isoprenaline, ephedrine and noradrenaline because of potential side effects (Table 1.3). Since aerosol administration of selective beta$_2$ agonists does not induce cardiovascular effects at therapeutic doses it cannot be considered to be an ergogenic aid. Administration of these drugs by any route other than aerosol is prohibited.

2. Methyl xanthines. Both theophylline and aminophylline (the soluble ethylenediamine-derivative of theophylline) are related to caffeine. They constitute the second line of bronchodilator therapy because they must be given orally or intravenously as the risk of side effects is much greater than with selective beta$_2$ agonists. The dose should be adjusted to provide a therapeutic plasma theophylline concentration of 10–20 μg/ml. Although the absolute threshold varies between individuals, both the frequency and severity of side effects increases with the plasma concentration. Thus 15 μg/ml is associated with nausea, vomiting, abdominal pains, headache, nervousness and muscle tremor. Plasma concentrations between 20 and 40 μg/ml can cause convulsions and ventricular arrhythmias increasing in severity from tachycardia to fibrillation and ultimately cardiac arrest. Sustained-release tablets are now the formulation of choice because they have reduced the fluctuations in plasma concentrations of theophylline and hence have reduced the incidence of side effects. Cardiovascular side effects are associated more with theophylline and central nervous system side effects with caffeine. Caffeine is banned by the IOC if the urinary concentration exceeds 12 μg/ml. In view of the considerable potential for the abuse of both the cardiovascular and CNS side effects of methyl xanthines, a decision to ban their use would seem to be eminently justifiable.

3. Anticholinergic drugs. The parasympathetic nervous system causes contraction of bronchial smooth muscle by the release of acetylcholine. Theoretically, therefore, anticholinergic drugs should be of benefit in the treatment of asthma. In practice, they have been of little use but they are indicated for the treatment of reversible airway obstruction in the chronic bronchitic. Inhaled ipratropium bromide, which is a quaternary derivative of atropine, is a useful alternative for individuals who cannot tolerate or respond to beta$_2$ agonists. It has a slow onset time (30–60 min) and is active for 3–4 hours. It may be better for the prevention than for the relief of symptoms. The side effects are those associated with antagonism of the parasympathetic

nervous system such as dry mouth, urinary retention and constipation. It should not be given to children under 3 years because
thickening of the bronchial secretions may block the constricted
airways. The IOC permits the use of ipratropium bromide for the
treatment of asthma.

Exercise-induced asthma

Exercise-induced asthma (EIA) can be defined as large changes in
airway resistance induced by standardized exercise (Bundgaard, 1985).
It is, perhaps, more appropriate to think of it as post-exercise
bronchoconstriction because the maximum decrease in peak expiratory
flow rate (PEFR) and forced expiratory volume in first sec (FEV_1) occurs
between 15 and 20 minutes after the excercise has been completed. It
should not be confused with, nor used as an excuse for, the breathless-
ness that occurs during exercise! The ventilatory changes in EIA are
identical to those observed during a spontaneous asthma attack, i.e.
decreased tidal volume, PEFR, FEV_1, FVC (forced vital capacity) and
increased residual volume (RV).

Exercise of less than 1 minute duration actually increases FEV_1 in the
asthmatic. After 1 minute the FEV_1 decreases. The severity of the
bronchoconstriction is decreased by warm temperature and high
humidity. Cooling and drying of the airways are thought to be
responsible for EIA. Between 50 and 70% of asthmatics experience
bronchoconstriction after exercise. Non-asthmatics are not affected in
this way. The severity of the bronchoconstriction is directly related to
the degree of hyperpnoea and hence to the duration and intensity of the
workload. Failure to appreciate the interaction between these variables
has lead to misconceptions about the relative benefits of swimming *vis à
vis* other sporting activities. When the intensity of work is standardized,
there is no difference between the asthma induced by swimming and
that which is produced by cycling, walking or running. There is no
diurnal variation in the response to exercise. The possibility of increased
sensitivity during the pollen season is controversial (Bundgaard, 1985).

Treatment of exercise-induced asthma

The aim of treatment is to prevent the asthmatic attack and to normalize
the exercise tolerance of the individual. $Beta_2$ agonists and SCG are the
most effective therapies.

1. Beta$_2$ agonists. These drugs are the most effective prophylactic treatment of EIA. Inhalation is preferable to oral administration because of greater speed of onset and reduced side effects. Terbutaline, salbutamol, rimiterol, orciprenaline and fenoterol have all been shown to provide effective prophylactic treatment of EIA. However, only the first four drugs are permitted by the IOC.
2. Sodium cromoglycate. SCG is not as effective as beta$_2$ agonists in the prevention of EIA. Children who suffer from extrinsic asthma are most likely to show a reduction in EIA after pre-treatment with SCG. It should be administered 30 minutes before the start of exercise. There is no significant difference between the efficacy of dry powder, aerosol or nebulised SCG.
3. Methyl xanthines. Theophylline in plasma concentrations of 10 –24 μg/ml afforded incomplete protection in a group of 12 child asthmatics (Bundgaard, 1985). In two other studies, theophylline relieved the symptoms of EIA but did not prevent EIA from occurring. The greater risk of cardiovascular side effects from theophylline than from either inhaled beta$_2$ agonists or SCG would relegate theophylline to the third line of therapy for EIA. Theophylline is not banned by the IOC but perhaps this should be reviewed because of the well documented CNS and cardiovascular effects of doses in excess of the therapeutic range.
4. Steroids. Single doses of inhaled steroids do not afford protection against EIA. A 4-week trial of inhaled betamethasone valerate produced a significant improvement in EIA but this may have been related to better base-line control of asthma. Inhaled budesonide twice a day for 4 weeks produced a significant improvement in resting pulmonary function and in the benefit derived from pre-exercise aerosol terbutaline. This is interpreted as support for the hypothesis that the benefit to be derived from aerosol steroids is in the general management of asthma (Fitch, 1986).
5. Anticholinergic drugs. These drugs are of relatively minor importance in the treatment of EIA. Bronchodilatation produced by inhalation of 0.5 mg ipratropium bromide was equal to that of a beta$_2$ agonist but was not effective against EIA (Bundgaard, 1985). Perhaps most significantly, there have been two studies which have demonstrated a synergistic effect between SCG and ipratropium bromide in the treatment of EIA (Bundgaard, 1985). However, ipratropium bromide alone does not compare with beta$_2$ agonists in either the prevention or the reversal of EIA.

Treatment of coughs and colds

There are many preparations which can be bought over the counter (OTC) for the treatment of coughs and colds. Very often they contain more than one active component, some of which are banned by the IOC, e.g. sympathomimetics and narcotic analgesics. Therefore, great care must be taken by the sportsperson when purchasing a cough or cold remedy for consumption during the competition season.

Cough is a protective reflex which is initiated by either mechanical or chemical stimulation of the oral pharynx, larynx, trachea or bronchi. It is designed to remove mucus from the upper respiratory tract (URT). Most commonly it is a symptom of a self-limiting URT infection which will normally resolve, without treatment, within 3–4 days. Antibiotics are of no value because the infection is normally viral and not bacterial. Less frequently it is a symptom of serious disease of the respiratory tract but this is unlikely to be relevant to an individual who is participating in aerobic exercise.

The important therapeutic distinction is between productive and non-productive coughs. A productive cough is normally caused by a bacterial infection and requires antibiotic therapy as well as antitussive therapy. A non-productive cough is normally caused by a viral infection of the throat and often marks the onset of a cold. Other causes of coughing include bronchoconstriction (in asthmatics), drainage of excess mucus from the nasopharynx (particularly when lying down) and tenacious mucus which cannot be moved adequately by the action of cilia on the respiratory epithelium.

The major groups of antitussive drugs are:

1. Cough suppressants – narcotic analgesics and antihistamines.
2. Expectorants.
3. Demulcents.
4. Vasoconstrictors.
5. Bronchodilators.

Cough suppressants

Narcotic analgesics suppress coughs by inhibiting the cough centre in the medulla oblongata in the brainstem. Pholcodine and dextromethorphan are preferable to codeine and morphine because they cause less constipation and respiratory depression. They are present in many OTC preparations. Pholcodine should be avoided because its use is banned by the IOC. Dextromethorphan was removed from the banned list in July 1986.

Antihistamines reduce coughing by two mechanisms. Firstly, they have a central suppressant action and secondly, their anticholinergic action reduces the rate of mucus secretion. They are not banned by the IOC. Both narcotic analgesics and antihistamines can cause drowsiness.

Expectorants

These increase the volume and decrease the viscosity of respiratory mucus. They are emetics, i.e. they cause vomiting at high concentrations. At sub-emetic doses they are thought to irritate the gastric mucosa which in turn stimulates secretion of respiratory mucus by a vagal reflex. Expectorants are often dismissed as little more than harmless placebos. This is most certainly not the case. Expectorants such as squill and ipecacuanha can be cardiotoxic in patients with renal impairment, whilst iodides can cause hyperthyroidism and are contraindicated in pregnancy. Therefore, it is important to define those circumstances in which their use would be indicated. Thick tenacious mucus that cannot be cleared by coughing is a feature of bacterial infections of the lower respiratory tract not of viral infections of the upper respiratory tract. The former require antibiotic therapy in which case an expectorant may be prescribed by a doctor rather than sold over the counter by a pharmacist. Steam is an excellent expectorant.

Demulcents

Demulcents substitute for the natural function of the mucus, i.e. a mechanical barrier which coats and protects the epithelium of the respiratory tract. Viral infections destroy epithelial cells which contribute to the production of mucus. Hence there is less mucus to protect the inflamed mucosa. A dry, persistant cough exacerbates the removal of cells and should be stopped. Demulcents are very effective in preventing dry, non-productive coughs. Simple linctus, syrups and lozenges containing glycerin (glycerol), honey and lemon are widely available. Some lozenges also contain a local anaesthetic (benzocaine) or an antibacterial agent (cetylpyridinium) which may be advantageous for a particularly troublesome cough. Note that demulcents are only effective in those areas that they can reach, i.e. the oral pharynx and larynx. However, they are often all that is needed to treat a dry, non-productive cough caused by a self-limiting viral infection and they are quite safe.

Vasoconstrictors

Selective alpha$_1$ agonists phenylephrine, phenylpropanolamine (PPA), oxymetazoline and xylometazoline will reduce nasal secretions by decreasing blood flow to the respiratory mucosa. These drugs are described as decongestants. However, they may increase the viscosity of respiratory secretions and cause congestion in some individuals. They are most effective in preventing the runny nose (rhinnorrhoea) that accompanies the common cold (coryzal syndrome), and which makes the external nares and alae so sore.

Both phenylephrine and PPA are powerful, orally active, vasoconstrictors. PPA is banned in the USA because of several reports of acute hypertensive episodes in some normal individuals after as little as a single oral dose of 25 mg, a concentration which is contained in many OTC preparations. In view of the CNS and CVS side effects of oral preparations (see above), and because they cannot be targeted to the desired site of action, topical formulations, i.e. drops or sprays, are the preferred route of administration. Oxymetazoline and xylometazoline, which are potent and long-acting vasoconstrictors, need only be applied twice daily. They are the drugs of choice for the treatment of rhinnorrhoea. Once again it should be borne in mind that alpha-adrenoceptor agonists, being sympathomimetics, are banned by the IOC with the exception of oxymetazoline spray.

Bronchodilators

Selective beta$_2$ agonists are not used in any cough or cold medicines. Instead either a non-selective sympathomimetic (ephedrine or pseudo-ephedrine) or a xanthine, e.g. caffeine or theophylline, is used as a bronchodilator. Both non-selective beta agonists and caffeine (when the plasma concentration exceeds 15 μg/ml) are banned by the IOC. Bronchodilators are only appropriate for lower respiratory tract infections where there is bronchoconstriction or a wheeze. Bronchodilators are of no relevance to the treatment of a congested pharynx, larynx or nasal cavity. Preparations which include a bronchodilator cannot be recommended to the sportsperson.

Table 1.4 Some of the more common drugs contained in OTC cough and cold medicines

Class of drug	Examples
Narcotic analgesics*	Codeine Pholcodine Morphine Dextromethorphan
Non-narcotic analgesics	Acetylsalicylic acid (aspirin) Paracetamol
Antihistamines	Promethazine Chlorpheniramine Dipheniramine Bromopheniramine Tripolidine
Sympathomimetics*	Ephedrine Pseudoephedrine Phenylephrine Phenylpropanolamine (PPA) Oxymetazoline Xylometazoline
Xanthines	Caffeine Theophylline
Expectorants	Ammonium citrate Sodium citrate Ipecacuanha Squill Guaiphenesin

* Banned by the IOC.

Self help

The following are recommendations for self-treatment of coughs and colds:

1. Hydration. This will prevent dehydration when there is copious secretion and will aid expectoration when a cough is non-productive.
2. Since a cough is designed to remove mucus, a productive cough should *never* be suppressed. A decongestant may be used if the

secretions are watery and arising from the nasopharynx. A purulent secretion requires antibiotic therapy from a medical practitioner.

3. A cough should only be suppressed when it is dry and non-productive (often a prelude to a viral infection of the upper respiratory tract). However, demulcents are preferable to cough suppressants if the cause is an inflamed throat because they have no side effects and they are not banned by the IOC.

4. Many cough and cold remedies cannot be recommended because they contain irrational combinations of either cough suppressants and expectorants and antihistamines or decongestants and expectorants. Some compound preparations contain sub-therapeutic concentrations of the active ingredients. Many of the active constituents are banned by the IOC (Table 1.4). Therefore, always attempt to purchase a product with a single active constituent. Always check the list of active drugs in the pharmaceutical preparation against the list of banned drugs that is readily available. If in doubt about either the mode of action or the type of drug and whether it is likely to be banned, ask a pharmacist and then your coach. The major groups of drugs which are contained in OTC cough and cold medicines are summarized in Table 1.4.

1.4 Adrenergic antagonists

1.4.1 BETA ANTAGONISTS (BETA BLOCKERS)

Beta-antagonists block beta-adrenoceptors and hence prevent adrenaline and noradrenaline from exerting those effects which are beta-receptor mediated. The significance of this group of drugs to the sportsperson is twofold. Firstly, they are being prescribed increasingly for a wide variety of clinical conditions and people may be unaware of the effects that this will have upon their ability to perform exercise. Secondly, beta blockers are developing into a major group of drugs of abuse in sport, principally because of their ability to reduce the effects of anxiety.

Beta receptors are widely distributed throughout the tissues and organs of the body, e.g. heart, blood vessels, bronchi, eyes, liver, pancreas and gastrointestinal tract, adipose tissue, skeletal muscle and the brain as indicated in Table 1.1. They can be subdivided into $beta_1$ and $beta_2$ receptors. $Beta_1$ receptors predominate in the heart. They also

Table 1.5 The cardioselectivity and lipid solubility of some commonly used beta blockers

Beta blocker	Cardioselectivity	Lipid solubility
Propranolol	−	+
Acebutolol	+/−	+
Oxprenolol	−	+
Metoprolol	+	+
Timolol	−	−
Pindolol	−	−
Sotalol	−	−
Betaxolol	+	−
Nadolol	−	−
Atenolol	+	−

stimulate lipolysis in adipose tissue thus increasing the plasma concentration of free fatty acids (FFA) which can be metabolized by skeletal muscle. Beta$_2$ receptors cause bronchodilation, release insulin from the pancreas and stimulate glycogenolysis in liver and skeletal muscle. These last three effects all increase glucose availability to the exercising muscle. Hence a beta$_2$ antagonist would be expected to decrease endurance capability. All beta blockers block beta$_1$ receptors. Those antagonists with a greater affinity for beta$_1$ as opposed to beta$_2$ receptors are described as cardioselective. Cardioselectivity is lost as the dose is increased so the distinction may not be of great therapeutic significance (Hudson, 1985). Table 1.5 indicates the cardioselectivity of some common beta blockers.

Clinical uses of beta blockers

Beta blockers are used to treat a variety of conditions including cardiac arrhythmias, glaucoma, hyperthyroidism, migraine and essential tremor. Most commonly they are used to treat angina pectoris and hypertension.

Angina pectoris is a symptom of coronary artery disease. It is the pain associated with reduced oxygen availability to, or ischaemia of, the myocardium. This means that the demand for oxygen from the myocardium is not matched by the supply of blood, i.e. coronary blood flow is inadequate. There are two causes of angina – effort and vasospasm. The management of angina involves reduction of risk factors (e.g. obesity, cigarette smoking, lack of exercise, hyperlipidaemia and hypertension) and drug treatment.

Organic nitrates are the first line treatment of angina. A significant proportion of patients cannot tolerate nitrates because they cause severe headaches. Beta blockers are the second choice for the treatment of angina of effort but are less effective in treating angina caused by vasospasm (unstable angina or Prinzmetal's syndrome). The third group of anti-anginal drugs, calcium antagonists, are indicated for unstable angina but are frequently used to treat angina of effort.

Hypertension (high blood pressure) is defined as a resting systolic and/or diastolic pressure exceeding the 95th percentile on at least three separate occasions (Walther and Tifft, 1985).

Anti-hypertensive and anti-anginal effects of beta blockers

Beta blockers affect both the heart and blood vessels. They reduce the work of the heart and hence its oxygen demand by reducing heart rate, myocardial contractility and peripheral resistance. A reduction in heart rate *per se* improves coronary blood flow because the latter occurs mainly during diastole which increases in duration as heart rate decreases. The dose of beta blocker is adjusted for each individual to obtain a resting heart rate of 50–60/min which should give a maximum rate of 100–120/min. The reductions in heart rate and myocardial contractility reduce cardiac output and hence arterial blood pressure. These anti-hypertensive effects of beta blockers are evident within 2 days to 2 weeks of regular treatment (Hudson, 1985). Subsequently, stroke volume may increase as peripheral resistance decreases and cardiac output at rest returns to pre-treatment values. However, blood pressure is still reduced because of the decrease in peripheral resistance. The decrease in peripheral resistance reduces the after-load against which the heart must pump. This in turn reduces the work of the heart and the oxygen requirement of the myocardium. The way in which beta blockers decrease peripheral resistance is controversial. Decreased renin release from the kidneys, noradrenaline release from post-ganglionic sympathetic nerve terminals and central sympathetic nervous system activity have been cited as possible explanations. However, some would maintain that beta blockers increase peripheral resistance (Walther and Tifft, 1985) by exposing alpha-receptor mediated vasoconstriction (Powles, 1981).

Beta blockers and exercise

Effects upon the cardiovascular and respiratory systems

Exercise in healthy individuals increases heart rate, myocardial contractility, stroke volume, cardiac output, $\dot{V}O_2$ and a-$\bar{v}O_2$ difference. Antagonism of beta$_1$-receptors in the heart reduces heart rate and myocardial contractility at rest. This effect is absent or negligible in elite athletes with very low resting heart rates (Tesch, 1985). During sub-maximal exercise in healthy subjects, beta blockers decrease heart rate, systolic blood pressure and cardiac output, increase stroke volume and a-$\bar{v}O_2$ difference, and have no significant effect upon diastolic blood pressure, ventilation and $\dot{V}O_2$. Stroke volume is increased at both submaximal and maximal work loads. This effect is not related to cardioselectivity.

Maximum cardiac output is decreased by beta blockers but the decrease is less than the decrease in maximum heart rate because of the compensatory rise in stroke volume. Once again this effect is not related to cardioselectivity. The majority of reports suggest that oxygen uptake at sub-maximal work loads is unaffected by beta blockade. However, $\dot{V}O_2$ max. is reduced by beta blockade. A 30% reduction in heart rate causes a 10–15% reduction in $\dot{V}O_2$ max. in patients and also in trained and untrained individuals. Such a decrease can be obtained after a single dose of propranolol or metoprolol (Tesch, 1985). The effects are dose related. The reported effects upon $\dot{V}O_2$ max. vary between a decrease and no significant difference. This may be due to the control $\dot{V}O_2$ max. of the subjects before beta blockade. Thus, beta blockade had little effect upon $\dot{V}O_2$ max. in subjects whose control or unblocked $\dot{V}O_2$ max. was < 50 ml/kg/min but caused a significant reduction in $\dot{V}O_2$ max. in individuals whose control $\dot{V}O_2$ max. was > 50 ml/kg/min. The decrease in $\dot{V}O_2$ max. did not correlate well (r = 0.42) with the decrease in heart rate for the group as a whole. However, when the subjects were divided into three sub-groups on the basis of their unblocked $\dot{V}O_2$ max., the correlation between the decrease in heart rate and that in $\dot{V}O_2$ max. increased as the unblocked $\dot{V}O_2$ max. increased. (Wilmore et al., 1985). The authors suggest that those subjects with an unblocked $\dot{V}O_2$ max. of < 50 ml/kg/min can compensate for a decrease in heart rate by increasing stroke volume and a-$\bar{v}O_2$ difference. However, those subjects with a control $\dot{V}O_2$ max. > 50 ml/kg/min will be operating at maximum stroke volume and a-$\bar{v}O_2$ difference and therefore cannot compensate adequately for the decrease in heart rate. There was no apparent significant difference between the effects of a cardioselective beta blocker (atenolol) and those of the two non-selective beta blockers (propranolol and sotalol). Rather surprisingly, propranolol tended to produce a greater decrease in $\dot{V}O_2$ max. than did atenolol (Wilmore *et al.*, 1985).

Effects upon metabolism

Beta blockers do not affect muscle strength, power, speed of contraction or work capacity (Tesch, 1985). However, as indicated earlier, they do have profound effects upon metabolism and energy availability. Antagonism of $beta_2$ receptors reduces energy availability in skeletal muscle by three mechanisms. Firstly, it reduces the release of insulin from the beta cells in the Islets of Langerhans in the pancreas. Secondly, it reduces glycogenolysis in the liver which can lead to hypoglycaemia. Non-selective beta blockers cause a greater reduction in blood glucose levels at submaximal work loads than do selective $beta_1$ blockers. Thirdly, it reduces glycogenolysis in skeletal muscle so that less glucose is liberated from intramuscular glycogen stores. In addition, $beta_1$ selective blockers reduce lipolysis in adipose tissue and hence the concentration of free fatty acids (FFA) in the blood. These effects will be unimportant in explosive anaerobic events but will limit performance in endurance events. The ability to sustain submaximal work is reduced by beta blockers. The time to exhaustion on either a treadmill or a bicycle is reduced by beta blockade. Non-selective beta blockers (e.g. propranolol) inhibit muscle lipolysis and glycogenolysis more than cardioselective beta blockers (e.g. metoprolol) so they have a greater inhibitory effect upon time to exhaustion. However, metoprolol (a cardioselective beta blocker) inhibits lipolysis more than glycogenolysis so that muscle glycogen is reduced more rapidly in metoprolol-treated than in control subjects (Allen *et al.*, 1984).

Effects upon psychomotor function

Non-selective beta blockers, e.g. propranolol, give effective relief of the physical symptoms of anxiety, e.g. palpitations, tremor, facial flushing and diarrhoea. The ability of a beta blocker to relieve the symptoms of anxiety increases with its lipophilicity which determines the rate at which it can cross the blood–brain barrier. Reduction in these physical symptoms *per se*, reduces the state of anxiety. However, the more lipophilic beta blockers (Table 1.5) are also more likely to cause insomnia, nightmares and depression which are the centrally-mediated undesirable side effects of beta blockers. Also, they preferentially inhibit lipolysis in adipose tissue. Essential tremor responds well to non-selective beta antagonists.

Side effects of treatment with beta blockers

1. Bronchospasm. Blockade of beta$_2$ receptors may precipitate bronchoconstriction in either asthmatics or chronic bronchitics.
2. Heart failure. Inhibition of sympathetic tone to the heart may precipitate cardiac failure in individuals with compromised cardiac function. The effect is enhanced by interaction with other cardiodepressant drugs, e.g. verapamil and lignocaine.
3. Heart block. Since these drugs are used to slow heart rate, they cannot be given to individuals who have an existing bradycardia due to a conduction defect, e.g. 2nd or 3rd degree heart block.
4. Cold extremities. Beta blockers reduce vasodilatation and reveal alpha receptor mediated vasoconstriction. This will aggrevate peripheral vascular disease and may lead to intermittent claudication or to Raynaud's disease.
5. Destabilization of diabetes mellitus. Beta blockers can decrease glucose tolerance and reduce the response to hypoglycaemia in diabetics. This effect is more marked with cardioselective beta blockers. However, even these drugs are contraindicated for diabetics who suffer from frequent hypoglycaemic episodes. Beta blockers do not induce diabetes in normal subjects.
6. Fatigue is a common side effect of the more lipophilic beta blockers. Atenolol, which is both cardioselective and only weakly lipophilic, is the beta blocker of choice in this case. A programme of exercise will often alleviate the symptoms of fatigue whilst at the same time improving cardiovascular function. Moreover, the symptoms of fatigue tend to decrease with time as the body accommodates to the effects of beta blockade.

Effects of beta blockade on the responses to exercise of hypertensive and ischaemic heart disease patients

HYPERTENSIVE SUBJECTS
Beta blockers will impair performance of endurance exercise (30 min duration) in patients with asymptomatic, uncomplicated hypertension.

Non-selective beta-blockers will also decrease the response to a training programme probably because of the deleterious effects upon carbohydrate and lipid metabolism. The effects of the beta blocker are dose related with differences in sensitivity between individuals. The effects upon $\dot{V}O_2$ max. are inconclusive (Allen *et al.*, 1984).

ISCHAEMIC HEART DISEASE (IHD) SUBJECTS

Beta blockers will facilitate an initial increase in exercise capacity in IHD subjects because of the improvement in the availability of oxygen to the myocardium at rest. Any improvement in the symptoms of exercise-induced angina should be used to encourage the subject to undertake an exercise programme which will augment the improvement in cardiovascular status. The training effect will be limited by the inhibitory effects of the beta blocker upon maximal heart rate and muscle metabolism. However, long-term treatment with a selective $beta_1$ antagonist will have more of a favourable effect upon plasma lipids and less of an inhibitory effect upon exercise-induced changes in plasma lipids than will non-selective blockade. Whether the cardioselective blocker should be more or less lipophilic remains the subject of conjecture (Tesch, 1985). Objective assessment of the interaction between exercise and beta blockade in IHD is difficult because of the criteria (changes in heart rate and $\dot{V}O_2$ max.) that are normally used to assess responses to a training programme. Beta blockade, *per se*, reduces heart rate and limitation of exercise testing by the onset of symptoms of angina introduces an element of subjectivity.

It should be remembered that beta blockade affects the physiological and biochemical responses to exercise so that the warm-up and cool-down periods need to be increased accordingly. An increase in warm-up will permit a gradual increase in both muscle blood flow (thus reducing anaerobic metabolism) and lipolysis. A longer cool-down period will reduce the light-headedness and fainting that can result from post-exercise hypotension (Allen *et al.*, 1984).

Potential for abuse of beta blockers

Beta blockers cannot be recommended for individuals who wish to participate in those events in which sub-maximal and maximal oxygen utilization is of prime importance (Walther and Tifft, 1985).

The major area of potential abuse for beta blockers lies in those events in which motor skills can be affected by muscle tremor caused by anxiety. Two studies have demonstrated a significant improvement in performance of some ski jumpers, bowlers and pistol-shooters after administration of the non-selective, lipophilic, beta blocker oxprenolol (40 mg/day). Those competitors who did demonstrate an improved performance during beta blockade were still able to increase heart rate significantly whereas those whose performance did not improve were unable to demonstrate an increase in heart rate (Tesch, 1985). Hence cardioselective beta blockers would be contraindicated. Quite rightly, this point should be of academic interest as the Olympic Committee plan to ban the use of beta blockers for the 1988 Olympics.

1.4.2 ALPHA ANTAGONISTS (ALPHA BLOCKERS)

These drugs are used in the treatment of hypertension and other vascular disorders. They produce their therapeutic effects by causing dilatation of peripheral blood vessels following blockade of alpha adrenoceptors.

Alpha adrenoceptors are subdivided into alpha$_1$ and alpha$_2$ adrenoceptors. The alpha$_2$ adrenoceptors are located pre-synaptically, that is on the membrane of sympathetic nerve endings. Their physiological function is to control the amount of the neurotransmitter, noradrenaline, released from the nerve endings when the nerves are stimulated. Some of the released noradrenaline acts upon these pre-synaptic alpha$_2$ adrenoceptors thereby inhibiting further release of noradrenaline. This is a negative feedback mechanism.

Alpha$_1$ adrenoceptors are found post-synaptically on the membranes of the smooth muscle within the tissue being innervated by the sympathetic nerves. It is through these alpha$_1$ adrenoceptors that the neurotransmitter, noradrenaline, interacts to cause contraction of the smooth muscle. An important example of this is seen within the arterial blood vessels. Sympathetic nerve stimulation leads to noradrenaline release which in turn acts on the alpha$_1$ adrenoceptors in the smooth muscle of the walls of the arterioles resulting in vasoconstriction. This vasoconstriction or narrowing of the arterioles is responsible for maintaining normal blood pressure and is known as sympathetic tone.

Hypertension (elevated blood pressure) can result from an identifiable cause, removal of which abolishes the hypertension. However, the majority of cases of hypertension are of unknown origin and are referred to as essential hypertension. Treatment of this condition is therefore symptomatic, in that the underlying cause cannot be treated as it is unknown. Consequently, patients suffering from essential hypertension are normally on drug therapy for life. This can present complications for hypertensives who are otherwise fit and well and who may therefore participate in a wide variety of sports.

There are several groups of drugs which are used to treat hypertensive patients and which have widely differing modes of action. The most widely prescribed drugs are diuretics and beta blockers because of their pharmacological effectiveness and their relatively low incidence of side effects at the therapeutic dose levels used. Other groups of drugs include vasodilators, calcium antagonists, angiotensin converting enzyme inhibitors and centrally acting drugs. The vasodilator group of drugs includes the alpha blockers.

In the past, alpha blockers such as phentolamine, tolazoline and phenoxybenzamine were used to treat hypertension but caused two major side effects – postural hypotension manifested by a tendency towards dizziness on standing up and tachycardia or rapid heart rate. More recently a second generation of alpha blockers has emerged which have a selective action on alpha$_1$ adrenoceptors. Prazosin and indoramin are members of this group of selective alpha blockers in current therapeutic use.

The advantage of alpha$_1$ selectivity lies in the fact that alpha$_1$ adrenoceptors are occupied, thereby preventing the vasoconstrictor action of noradrenaline, released from the sympathetic nerves. The resultant vasodilatation leads to a decrease in blood pressure. With non-selective alpha blockers, the pre-synaptic alpha$_2$ adrenoceptors are also blocked. Therefore, the negative feedback mechanism is inhibited and a greater amount of noradrenaline is released from sympathetic nerve endings. In tissues where the post-synaptic receptors are of the alpha$_1$ type this does not matter as these are protected by the alpha blocker. However, where the post-synaptic receptors are of the beta type there is no protection against the increased noradrenaline released. This is the case in the heart and accounts for the tachycardia associated with non-selective alpha blockers. Prazosin and indoramin have a reduced affinity for alpha$_2$ adrenoceptors; hence, the incidence of tachycardia with these drugs is greatly diminished.

The selective alpha blockers are also less likely to dilate venous blood vessels which carry the blood back to the heart. Venous return is, therefore, improved and this helps to reduce the incidence of postural hypotension.

Alpha blockers are not drugs of abuse in sport nor have there been any reports of their adverse effects in exercise performance. It is pertinent to note that patients who are hypertensive often experience no symptoms. All antihypertensive drugs, however, induce various degrees of side effects. A patient may therefore end up with a poorer quality of life on antihypertensive drugs compared with when their hypertension was untreated. It must be stressed, however, that untreated hypertension can lead to more serious diseases such as stroke with a high risk of mortality. Long-term exercise has been proposed as an alternative to drug therapy for reducing blood pressure in hypertensives. Unfortunately, a recent study by Kenney and Zambaski (1984) provided equivocal evidence and led them to conclude that the effect of training on the chronic high blood pressure of hypertensives is still unclear.

1.5 References

Allen, C. J., Craven, M. A., Rosenbloom, D., Sutton, J. R. (1984) Beta-blockade and exercise in normal subjects and patients with coronary artery disease. *Physician and Sports Medicine*, 12, 51–63.

Bundgaard, A. (1985) Exercise and the asthmatic. *Sports Medicine*, 2, 254–66.

Clark, T. J. H. (1983) *Steroids in Asthma. A Reappraisal in the Light of Inhalation Therapy.* Auckland ADIS Press, UK pp. 11–31, 46–60.

Clark, T. J. H. and Cochrane, G. M. (1984) *Bronchodilator Therapy: The Basis of Asthma and Chronic Obstructive Airways Disease Management.* Auckland ADIS Press, UK pp. 17–46.

Eisenstadt, W. S., Nicholas, S. S., Velick, G. and Enright, T. (1984) Allergic reactions to exercise. *Physician and Sports Medicine*, 12, 95–104.

Fitch, K. D. (1986) The use of anti-asthmatic drugs. Do they affect sports performance? *Sports Medicine*, 3, 136–50.

Hudson, S. A. (1985) Drug review: understanding β-blockers. *Pharmacy Update*, May, 74–7.

IOC (1988) Medical Controls Brochure.

Katzung, B. G. (1987) *Basic and Clinical Pharmacology*, 3rd edn. Lange, Los Altos, California.

Kenney, W. K. and Zambaski, E. J. (1984) Physical activity in human hypertension. A mechanisms approach. *Sports Medicine*, 1, 459–73.

Powles, A. C. P. (1981) The effects of drugs on the cardiovascular response to exercise. *Medicine and Science in Sports and Exercise*, 13, 252–8.

Tesch, P. A. (1985) Exercise performance and β-blockade. *Sports Medicine*, 2, 389–412.

Walther, R. J. and Tifft, C. P. (1985) High blood pressure in the competitive athlete: guidelines and recommendations. *Physician and Sports Medicine*, **13**, 93–114.

Wilmore, J. H., Joyner, M. J., Freund, B. J., Ewy, G. A. and Morton, A. R. (1985) Beta-blockade and response to exercise: influencing of training. *Physician and Sports Medicine*, **13**, 61–9.

2   Anabolic steroids

A. J. GEORGE

2.1 Summary

The conclusions reached in surveying anabolic steroid use in male and female athletes are that anabolic steroids probably do increase muscle bulk and body weight in all anabolic steroid takers but that increases in strength are certain to occur only in those undertaking regular training exercise. The long term side effects of anabolic steroids are severe and will depend on dosage and duration. In particular early death from cardiovascular disease, sterility in men and, in women, masculinization and possible fetal effects constitute the most serious hazards. It is likely that the full impact of pathological changes induced by anabolic steroids will not be apparent until the 1990s when those athletes who took large doses of anabolic steroid in the late 60s and early 70s, before the advent of controlling legislation, reach late middle age.

2.2 Introduction

For centuries, it was popularly believed that symptoms of ageing in men were caused by testicular failure. This stimulated a search for an active principle of the testicles which, when isolated, would restore sexual and mental vigour to ageing men. The testicular principle, which we now know is the male sex hormone testosterone, was first synthesized in 1935.

Experimental studies in both animals and humans soon showed that testosterone possessed both anabolic and androgenic actions. The androgenic actions of testosterones are those actions involving the development and maintenance of primary and secondary sexual characteristics while the anabolic actions consist of the positive effects

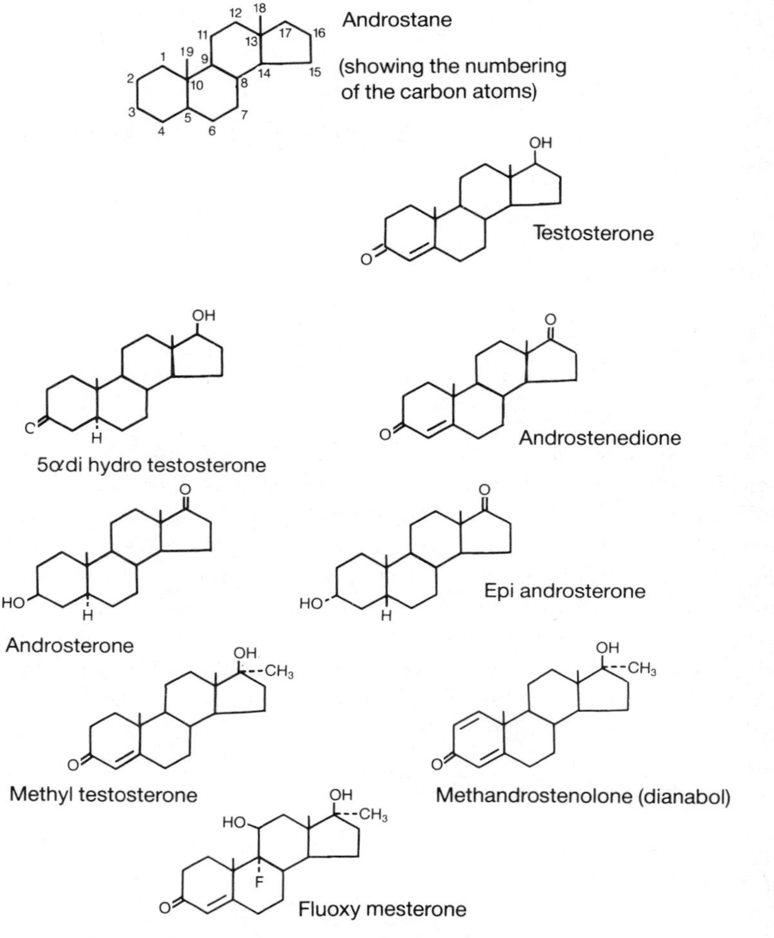

Figure 2.1 The structure of some androgens and anabolic steroids.

of testosterone in inhibiting urinary nitrogen loss and stimulating protein synthesis, particularly in skeletal muscle.

2.3 The testosterone family

Testosterone is a so-called C-19 steroid hormone. The steroid hormones are derived in the body from the substance cholesterol. The structure of testosterone is closely related to the steroid substance androstane and the structure of androstane is used as a reference when naming most of the compounds related to or derived from testosterone (Figure 2.1).

2.3.1 THE BIOCHEMISTRY AND PHYSIOLOGY OF TESTOSTERONE

Testosterone, the most important naturally occurring compound with androgen and anabolic activity is formed in the Leydig cells of the testis and also in the adrenal cortex. Adrenocortical and ovarian testosterone is important in women as it is responsible for some secondary sexual characteristics such as pubic and axillary hair growth and in some cases for its influence on sexuality. Mean testosterone production in men is approximately 8 mg/day of which 90–95% is produced by the testis and the remainder by the adrenal cortex. The testis also produces 5α dihydrotestosterone which is approximately equal in androgenic and anabolic activity to testosterone and also two compounds with much weaker biological activity: androstenedione and dehydroepiandrosterone. After puberty plasma testosterone levels are approximately 0.6 μg/dl in males and 0.03 μg/dl in women. Most (95%) of the testosterone in the blood is bound to protein mainly sexhormone-binding globulin (SHBG); 2–3% of testosterone remains free, i.e. unbound, while the remainder is bound to serum albumin.

Mode of action

Like most other steroid hormones testosterone produces its effect on tissues by altering cellular biochemistry in an interaction with the cell nucleus. Testosterone diffuses into the cell as it is lipid soluble and thus readily crosses cell membranes. It combines with a testosterone binding protein which transports it to the cell nucleus. Here the testosterone interacts with one or more specific binding sites and activates the synthesis of one or more proteins which may be either enzymes or structural proteins. In some tissues testosterone is first converted to 5α dihydrotestosterone (DHT) by the enzyme 5α reductase. The DHT is then transported to the nucleus and produces similar biochemical changes to those of testosterone. Parts of the hypothalamus, in some mammals, are capable of converting testosterone to oestradiol via the enzyme 'aromatase'. This has been suggested as one mechanism by which testosterone influences sexual activity in males and females in species such as the rat.

Metabolism

Apart from conversion to DHT in various testosterone sensitive tissues, testosterone is metabolized in the liver mainly to androstenedione and then to either androsterone or one of its two isomers, epiandrosterone or etiocholanone. All three metabolites are present in plasma and urine. Androsterone and epiandrosterone have weak androgenic activity, while etiocholanone has none. Some testosterone is converted in the testis to oestradiol. Significant amounts of oestradiol are also thought to be formed from testosterone in the brain.

2.3.2 THE PHYSIOLOGICAL ROLE OF TESTOSTERONE

Testosterone and its structurally related analogues possess androgenic and anabolic activity.

Androgenic effects

Testosterone is responsible for the development of primary sexual characteristics in males. Normally, in a genetically male fetus, i.e. one with the XY sex chromosome configuration, the embryonic testis begins to differentiate under the influence of H-Y antigen, the production of which is directed by the Y chromosome. As the male gonad differentiates, Leydig cells are formed which begin to secrete testosterone. Testosterone and a polypeptide factor, MRF (Mullerian regression factor) together stimulate the formation of the male genitalia. The external genitalia develop solely under the influence of testosterone. From birth until puberty the Leydig cells which secrete testosterone produce small amounts of testosterone. From the age of approximately 10 years, increased testosterone secretion occurs from the adrenal gland and then at puberty (11–14 years) an upsurge in testosterone secretion occurs principally from the testicular Leydig cells. The pubertal changes induced by this increase in testosterone are the secondary sexual characteristics which include changes in hair distribution, musculoskeletal configuration, genital size, psychic changes and induction of sperm production. The chronology of male puberty and adolescence has been described in detail by Tanner (1962) and the

Tanner Index provides a useful guide for the assessment of the progress of puberty, and the attainment of maturity.

Anabolic effects

The anabolic effects of testosterone and anabolic steroids are usually considered to be those promoting protein synthesis and muscle growth but they also include effects such as stimulation and inhibition of skeletal growth in the young. Attempts to produce purely anabolic, synthetic testosterone derivatives have been unsuccessful. It should be remembered that though the anabolic effects of the so-called anabolic steroids may be much greater than testosterone, all anabolic steroids also possess androgenic activity.

2.3.3 CLINICAL USES OF ANDROGENS/ANABOLIC STEROIDS

Replacement therapy in men

Anabolic steroids may be given to stimulate sexual development in cases of delayed puberty. The therapy is then withdrawn gradually once full sexual maturity is reached. They may also be given in cases where the testicles have been surgically removed either because of physical injury or because of a testicular tumour. In this case the replacement therapy must be continuous for life.

Gynaecological disorders

Anabolic steroids are occasionally used to treat gynaecological conditions in women, though long-term usage produces severe side effects such as erratic menstruation and the appearance of male secondary sexual characteristics. In the USA, they are sometimes used to suppress lactation after childbirth. They are also sometimes used to combat breast tumours in premenopausal women.

Protein anabolism

The initial use of anabolic steroids in the early 1940s was to inhibit the loss of protein and aid muscle regeneration after major surgery, and to stimulate muscle regeneration in debilitating disorders such as muscular dystrophy and diabetes. Many concentration camp survivors owe their early recovery from debilitation to the skilled use of dietary measures coupled with anabolic steroids.

Anaemia

Anabolic steroids are sometimes used in large doses to treat anaemias which have proved resistant to other therapies – this therapy is not recommended in women because of masculinizing side effects.

Osteoporosis

There is some evidence that combined oestrogen/androgen therapy is able to inhibit bone degeneration in this disorder.

Growth stimulation

Anabolic steroids may be used to increase growth in prepubertal boys who have failed to reach their expected height for their age. The treatment must be carried out under carefully controlled conditions so that early fission of the epiphyses does not occur.

2.3.4 SIDE EFFECTS OF ANDROGENS

Principally in women

These include acne, growth of facial hair, hoarsening or deepening of the voice. If the dose given is sufficient to suppress gonadotrophin secretion then menstrual irregularities will occur. Chronic, i.e. long-term treatment with androgens, as for example in mammary carcinoma, may produce the following side effects – male pattern baldness, prominent musculature and veins, and clitoral hypertrophy.

In children

Administration of androgens can cause stunting of growth, a side effect directly related to disturbance of normal bone growth and development. The enhancement of epiphyseal closure is a particularly persistent side effect which can be present up to 3 months after androgen withdrawal.

In males

Spermatogenesis is reduced by testosterone treatment with as little as 25 mg testosterone per day over a 6 week period. Anabolic steroids will produce the same effect, since they will suppress natural testosterone secretion. The inhibition of spermatogenesis may persist for many months after anabolic steroid withdrawal.

General side effects

Oedema

Oedema or water retention, related to the increased retention of sodium and chloride is a frequent side effect of short-term androgen administration. This may be the major contribution to the initial weight gain seen in athletes taking these drugs (see p. 66). Water and electrolyte gain is an unwanted side effect in all normal individuals but is particularly unhealthy in people with circulatory disorders or in those with a family background of such disorders.

Jaundice

This is a frequent side effect of anabolic steroid therapy and is caused mainly by reduced flow and retention of bile in the biliary capillaries of the hepatic lobules. Hepatic cell damage is not usually present. Those anabolic steroids with a 17α methyl group are most likely to cause jaundice.

Hepatic carcinoma

Patients who have received androgens and/or anabolic steroids for prolonged periods may develop hepatic carcinoma. This is particularly prevalent in people who have taken the 17α methyl testosterone derivatives.

2.4 Anabolic steroids and sport

The desire to increase sporting performance and athletic prowess by means other then physical training has been experienced for at least 2000 years. A recent review by Ryan (1981) quotes the observation of the Greeks that a high protein diet was essential for body building and athletic achievement. The Greeks of course knew nothing of protein structure or biosynthesis but they felt that by eating the flesh of a strong animal such as the ox, the athlete would gain strength himself. We have seen previously that one of the first therapeutic uses of anabolic steroids was in treating the protein loss and muscle wasting suffered by concentration camp victims. Following the publication of the results of these treatments it was natural that anabolic steroids should be used in an attempt to increase muscle strength in athletes. Many early studies on the effect of anabolic steroids often involved self administration and were necessarily anecdotal with no attempt at a scientific or controlled investigation of the effect of the steroid drugs. Several studies relied on subjective feelings and lacked any objective measure of increased strength or stamina. Also, side effects were never admitted to or were simply omitted from the results.

Subsequent studies, many of which were carried out in the late 1960s and early 1970s, were more scientifically based but often entirely contradictory in their results. In this section we will discuss what any physician, student or lay person would wish to know about the use of an anabolic steroid: does it work?; does it confer any advantage over normal training practices?; what are the side effects?; what are the long- and short-term consequences? In addition, the athlete needs to know whether the practice is ethical and the sports administrator how to discover whether anabolic steroids are being taken. Finally we will consider the future trends.

Whether anabolic steroid treatment 'works' is perhaps the most difficult question of all to answer satisfactorily since the known investigations which have been carried out are, in the main, poorly designed scientifically, clinically and statistically (Ryan, 1981). Increases in muscle strength are proportional to increases in the cross-sectional diameter of the muscles being trained but there is no way of showing conclusively *in vivo* that any increase in muscle diameter consists of increased muscle protein rather than increased content of water or fat. It is also apparent that different groups of athletes may wish to increase their muscle bulk for different purposes. For example, the American footballer or the wrestler may wish simply to increase his bulk and weight, whereas a weightlifter may want increased dynamic strength and the long distance runner may wish to accelerate muscle repair after an arduous and taxing run.

The first serious investigator of the question as to whether anabolic steroids work seems to be Ryan (1981) who reviewed a total of 37 studies between the years 1968 and 1977. He was confounded by the many different measurements being taken as indices of anabolic steroid activity. Some studies attempted to measure gains in strength of experimental subjects over controls, other studies measured the change in circumference of a limb. One study attempted to measure change in lean body mass. In 12 studies which claimed that athletes taking anabolic steroids gained in strength, the gains reported in these studies were often quite small. The majority of these 12 studies were not 'blind': that is either the investigator or the subject (or perhaps both!) knew when an active principle was being taken. In only five of the studies were protein supplements given and in none of the studies examined was there any dietary control over or at least a listing of the total protein and caloric intake for each subject. Other features of these studies were their poor design, in matching control and experimental subjects and there were also errors in calculating the results. Ryan then examined 13 other studies in which valid matching of controls and experiments had occurred. Ten of these 13 studies were double-blind (neither experimenter nor subject knew when an active substance was being administered), the control and experimental groups contained at least 6 subjects in each and the average period of experimentation was some 50% longer than in the early studies in which improvements were claimed. Also, in this second group of experiments, five different steroid drugs were investigated compared to only two in the earlier group. Ryan's conclusion from examining these two groups of studies was that there was no substantial evidence for an increase in lean muscle bulk or muscle strength in healthy young adult males receiving anabolic steroids. Comparison of these studies is difficult because the various parameters used to assess improvement in strength were not the same. Though the majority of studies assessed by Ryan measured changes in gross body weight and 'improvement' in standard strength tests, the other tests employed included $\dot{V}O_2$ max. limb circumference, lean body mass and 'changes in blood chemistry'. One reason for the variety of measurements used and a possible explanation for the lack of agreement in assessing anabolic steroid efficacy is that different athletic groups each sought different parameters for improvement. As I have mentioned before the American footballer or the wrestler may be seeking increased bulk, the weightlifter or thrower an increase in strength or perhaps both. Experiments with anabolic steroids since 1975, however, have tended to be more carefully carried out, better controlled and more sophisticated than those reviewed by Ryan. An example of a well-conducted trial is the frequently quoted study by Freed *et al.* (1975). In this study, six standard strength exercises were used as a measure of increased strength. The study was carried out over a 6 week period, in weightlifters who were given either 10 mg or 25 mg per day of methandienone. Drug treatment increased strength by 0.3–13% during the 6 week study while those taking placebo showed strength gains of 0.3–2.3%. Body weight increased only in the drug-treated athletes and those on the 25 mg dose showed no greater strength increase than those on 10 mg. A significant finding was that withdrawal of the anabolic steroid caused a loss of weight but no loss in strength gained, which suggested that anabolic steroid taking amongst athletes might be harder to detect since the drug could be withdrawn from an athlete well in advance of a meeting without a significant loss of performance thus allowing him to evade detection in any doping test. Further analysis of Freed's study shows that the doses of methandienone are some 75% lower than those claimed to be used by some athletes. It might have been more useful to tailor the dose of the drug to the athlete's initial body weight, i.e. calculate the dose in terms of mg/kg body weight and also to measure the actual free and bound plasma concentration of the drug. It is reasonable to conclude from Freed's work that only a proportion of people show a significant improvement in strength as a result of steroid treatment. Further studies should determine which types of athlete or individual 'benefit' from anabolic steroids. Another factor absent from the analyses of this and previous experiments is consideration of the subject's body build. The bodily changes induced by testosterone at puberty and indeed those that are produced *in utero* occur as a result of an interaction between testosterone and the individual's genetic 'constitution' or genotype. Thus, the individual emerging from puberty with a lean well-muscled body – the classical mesomorph somatotype – does so because of the expression of the genes controlling his muscularity rather than because he has higher testosterone levels than the more lightly-muscled ectomorph. Thus, only certain somatotypes may benefit from anabolic steroid treatment.

The importance of athletic experience and pre-training on the response of athletes to anabolic steroid treatment has been researched by Wright (1980). He noted that inexperienced weightlifters showed no increase in strength or lean muscle mass while simultaneously taking anabolic steroids and protein supplements and undergoing short-term training. In contrast, weightlifters who trained regularly, i.e. to nearly their maximum capacity, did show increased strength compared to their pre-treatment level. Though his results did not show consistent increases in strength among the steroid-treated trained athletes, Wright claimed to show that the trained athletes responded better to anabolic steroid treatment, a finding he could not explain adequately. However, the presence of a greater initial muscle mass in the trained athletes, before anabolic steroid treatment might have been a factor. Another possibility is that trained muscles are different, i.e. they may produce some endogenous factor which enhances anabolic steroid action. It is already known that the muscles of trained athletes can increase their uptake of glucose by the production of an endogenous factor and that regular exercise regimes increase the responsiveness of skeletal muscle to insulin.

If the results of these studies produce such inconsistent results why do athletes continue to take anabolic steroids? One possible explanation is that the steroid trials published so far are based on dose levels which, while medically and ethically acceptable, are considerably less than those commonly taken by athletes. This factor coupled with the necessity of pre-drug intensive training and a high protein diet might explain the failure of anabolic steroids to produce a consistent increase in strength and performance.

The importance of training before and during a period of steroid treatment is apparently emphasized in a sophisticated series of experiments carried out by Hervey and colleagues between 1976 and 1981, and reviewed recently by Hervey (1982). The experimental design involved the administration of the anabolic steroid dianabol 100 mg per day during one 6 week period and a placebo during the other 6 weeks. The two treatment periods (drug and placebo) were separated by a 6 week treatment-free period. The experiments were carried out double blind. All volunteers were athletes, one group being professional weightlifters. In each group body weight, body fat, body density and the fat and lean tissue proportion were measured.

The non-weightlifting group of athletes showed the same improvement in weightlifting performance and leg muscle strength during both placebo and drug administration periods. In the group containing experienced weightlifters there was a significant improvement during drug administration when compared to the placebo period. Both weightlifters and other athletes exhibited weight gain and increases in limb circumference. Although the weightlifters were heavier than their non-weightlifting counterparts the proportion of lean body mass was the same in both groups.

Hervey *et al.* (1981) concluded from these experiments that in athletes engaged in continuous hard-training regimes, anabolic steroids in the doses athletes claim to use cause an increase in muscle-strength and athletic performance. The experimental design could be criticized in that it is possible that those subjects taking the drug in the first 6 week period were not completely drug free at the start of the placebo period 6 weeks later. Thus, the residual effect of the steroid could have affected measurements during the placebo period of evaluation and could have masked any apparent differences between the placebo and treatment periods. In conclusion, anabolic steroids appear to increase muscle strength in those undertaking hard exercise and taking protein supplements.

If anabolic steroid administration does produce these increases in muscle strength, should this not be reflected in the progression of athletic records? Howard Payne analysed UK and world sporting records from 1950 to 1975. The trend in all the events analysed, namely the 10 000 metres, pole vault, discus and shot shows a steady improvement year by year without a sudden upsurge in any event. Thus, anabolic steroids cannot be shown to have significantly improved performances in field events nor in the 10 000 metres where competitors are erroneously assumed not to be steroid takers.

If even in the most careful experiments the positive effects of anabolic steroids are seen only in maximally exercising individuals, why is it that so many claims are made for them. One reason is possibly that steroids make them 'feel better'. Some athletes claim they feel more competitive and aggressive, others may feel they should run faster as they are on anabolic steroids. The increase in body weight and in circumference of leg and arm muscles may improve the athlete's self-image. Whether anabolic steroids enhance aggression or competitiveness is hard to assess. It is difficult to demonstrate conclusively that steroids or indeed testosterone are responsible for aggressiveness since many behaviours are probably learnt. It is quite likely that behaviour if it is hormonally influenced is imprinted soon after birth. However, both male and female sexual behaviour are strongly influenced by androgens (see Section 2.3.2).

If it is agreed that anabolic steroids do increase athletic performance, albeit in strictly defined circumstances, what advantages does it confer on the taker? Obvious advantages are that the steroid taker may have stronger muscles with greater endurance, and a greater body mass with which to endure impact in sports like rugby, ice hockey or wrestling. A further advantage conferred on the anabolic steroid taker is that their muscles and associated tissues may have greater reparative powers and so the athlete may be able to undertake more events in a short time. This observation has led to the increased use of steroids by both middle, long distance and marathon runners.

The original ideas that anabolic steroids simply simulate muscle growth need to be revised following the results of studies carried out in exercising individuals. From the results quoted previously, it is possible to deduce that anabolic steroids may simply allow more intense exercise to take place thus stimulating muscle growth. Again, it could be that muscle produces an endogenous factor which stimulates further muscle growth or that exercise induces increased production of the hormones such as insulin, growth hormone and somatomedins each of which is able to increase protein synthesis particularly in muscle. It is interesting that most major studies involving anabolic steroids, with the exception of that by Hervey *et al.* (1981), have failed to measure other hormones simultaneously. This study by Hervey *et al.* measured testosterone and cortisol during the treatment of athletes with methandienone. They showed that as testosterone was suppressed by methandienone treatment by the end of the experiment so plasma cortisol concentration rose. It is not clear whether this is the free, or total cortisol in the plasma, but the deduction made was that anabolic steroid effects are possibly mediated via a rise in cortisol concentration. The authors claimed that the puffy facial and thoracial features produced by anabolic steroids are similar to those occurring in Cushing's disease (CD) in which plasma cortisol is abnormally high as the result of either a pituitary or adrenocortical tumour producing adrenocortical overproduction of cortisol. There are many objections to this ingenious theory. The symptoms of CD and anabolic steroid administration are far from similar: CD patients have a characteristic moon face, abnormal fat distribution and distended abdomen; the limb muscles are thin and wasted, producing the characteristic 'lemon on sticks' appearance of CD sufferers. More importantly, the plasma cortisol levels in CD are much greater than those quoted by the authors at the end of their study. Cortisol and related compounds induce muscle wasting and a loss of amino acids (particularly alanine) into the blood and eventually to the liver. Finally, one would expect the increase in cortisol availability eventually to reduce cortisol secretion from the adrenal cortex via the normal negative feedback mechanisms.

2.4.1 ANABOLIC STEROID SIDE EFFECTS WITH
       PARTICULAR REFERENCE TO ATHLETES

In Section 2.3.4 the general side effects of anabolic steroids were
discussed. Of these side effects, some are of particular significance to
athletes taking steroids, namely cardiovascular side effects since
exercise imposes a particular stress on the cardiovascular system, and,
hepatic side effects because anabolic steroids, particularly those with
C_{17} alkyl substituents are suspected hepatic carcinogens in the doses in
which they are taken by athletes.

Cardiovascular effects

Anabolic steroids increase the rate of atherosclerosis in arteries and
arterioles and it is the secretion of testosterone in man which is thought
to be the major cause of the greater incidence of coronary heart disease
(CHD) in males compared to females in the under-50 age group.
Anabolic steroids have been shown to increase blood triglyceride and
cholesterol levels while decreasing the concentration of high-density
lipoproteins (HDL) which appear to provide protection against atherosclerosis. Several studies, especially the widely quoted Framlingham
study in the USA, have shown that a reduction of just 10% in the blood
concentration of HDL could increase the chances of coronary disease
by 25%. A more recent study by Costill, Pearson and Fink (1984) has
shown that in athletes taking anabolic steroids, HDL fell by 20% after
only 102 days of treatment, while cholesterol concentration was
unchanged. In normal males, 22% of cholesterol is in the form of HDL
while in steroid takers only 7.8% of cholesterol is found combined in
this way. There are several well-documented cases of CHD in
apparently fit, healthy athletes aged under 40, who have been taking
anabolic steroids (Goldman, 1984).

Salt and water retention

In the previous section, the effect of anabolic steroids on salt and water
retention was discussed in relation to steroid induced gains in body
weight and muscle circumference. The increase in salt and water
retention responsible for these changes has a deleterious effect on the
cardiovascular systems. Thus, the increased blood sodium concentration causes a rise in blood osmotic pressure; since sodium ions cannot
diffuse into cells they remain in the extra-cellular fluid and blood unless
excreted by the kidney, thus raising the osmotic pressure and withdraw-
ing water from the tissues. An expansion of the blood volume then

occurs which imposes an increased workload on the heart. The heart increases its output and the blood pressure rises. The increased sodium concentration may also directly stimulate vasoconstriction thus enhancing the hypertensive effect of the increased blood volume. Again the increased incidence of potentially fatal hypertension in athletes on anabolic steroids is well known (Goldman, 1984; Wright, 1980).

Carcinomas

The association between anabolic steroid administration and tumour formation, particularly of the liver and kidney, is now firmly established. Significant changes in liver biochemistry have been found in 80% of otherwise healthy athletes taking anabolic steroids but without any signs of liver disease. In 1965, a detailed case study was published linking the death of an anabolic steroid-taking athlete with hepatocellular cancer (HC). Since then 13 other athletes taking anabolic steroids have been shown to have HC and all were taking 17-alkylated androgens. A second more insidious liver pathology, petiocis hepatis was associated with anabolic steroids in 1977 (Goldman, 1984). In this disorder hepatic tissue degenerates and is replaced by blood filled spaces.

Anabolic steroids have also been suspected of causing death from Wilm's tumour of the kidney in two adult athletes. The tumour is very rare in post-adolescent individuals.

Fertility

In Section 2.3.1 it was noted that spermatogenesis in human males is under the control of gonadotrophins and testosterone. Administration of anabolic steroids caused inhibition of gonadotrophin secretion followed by inhibition of testosterone. Holma (1979) administered 15 mg methandienone to 15 well-trained athletes for 2 months. During the administration period sperm counts fell by 73% and in three individuals azoospermia (complete absence of sperm) was present. Even in those individuals with sperms present there was a 10% increase in the number of immotive sperms and 30% decrease in the number of motile sperms. Thus, fertility was severely reduced in males in this study which provides confirmation of many clinical reports of the same phenomena. Though it is obviously unethical to test this, much clinical data suggests that long-term anabolic steroid treatment may produce irreversible atrophy of testicular tissue suggesting that anabolic steroid-induced infertility might be permanent.

Effects on libido

The suppression of testosterone secretion in both males and females may well have effects on libido. As previously discussed, libido in males and females is thought to be influenced at least in part by testosterone. Thus, high levels of anabolic steroids in the blood suppress testosterone secretion and reduce libido.

Specific actions in female athletes

Considering the side effects mentioned in the introduction, people often wonder why female athletes should take anabolic steroids. The simple answer is that women's athletics is now as competitive as men's and that according to some reports, the effects of anabolic steroids on muscle strength and bulk in a training female athlete are considerably greater than in a male. This has been explained by the lower normal circulating level of testosterone in females as compared to men. Thus, some female athletes take anabolic steroids in the knowledge that they may produce greater muscle strength and bulk at the expense of irreversible change such as deepening of the voice and clitoral enlargement.

Tendons

Several researchers have noted the increased incidence of tendon damage in athletes taking anabolic steroids. This phenomenon has been explained in at least three different ways. Firstly, that the increase in muscle strength acquired by a course of steroids, plus training, produces a greater increase in muscle power than in tendon strength since tendons respond slowly to strength regimes and anabolic steroids have little or no effect on tendon strength. It is also thought that anabolic steroids have, in common with corticosteroids (such as cortisol), the ability to inhibit the formation of collagen – an important constituent of tendons and ligaments. Weightlifters taking anabolic steroids appear to be particularly prone to muscle and tendon injuries. This has been explained by apologists for anabolic steroids as evidence of greater weights being lifted. Sports doctors say it is the biochemical effects of anabolic steroids previously discussed, while others say that the increased aggressiveness and competitiveness induced by anabolic steroid administration causes athletes to attempt more and greater lifts with a more reckless attitude to the actual mechanics of the lifting.

2.5 The future

What further developments might there be concerning anabolic steroid administration? More stringent controls and methods of blood urine analysis may reduce the incidence of anabolic steroid taking. It is too soon to learn whether the proliferation of suspensions and disqualifications of the late 1970s and early 1980s has had any effect. It is certain that more subtle ways of drug-induced muscle building will be tried. For example, it is possible, by giving injections of luteinizing hormone (LH) to boost endogenous testosterone in a male. Though increasing LH doses would be needed, because of inhibitory testosterone feedback effects, this treatment could be held in reserve as a means of avoiding detection of anabolic steroid administration during the run-up to a major athletic event. Another method is to dispense with steroids altogether and to use growth hormone.

Growth hormone

Human growth hormone (hGH) is the next potential drug of abuse in sport and athletics. This prediction should be confined to Britain and the rest of Europe since the illicit use of hGH in the USA has already been described by Talyor (1985).

hGH is one the major hormones influencing growth and development in humans. Such is the complexity of human growth, a period extending from birth to the age of 20 years, that a very large number of hormones are involved, producing many complex interactions. Besides hGH the hormones, testosterone, oestradiol, cortisol, thyroxine and insulin have important roles at different stages of growth and development. The exact role of hGH in growth is difficult to evaluate exactly because of the many different developmental and metabolic processes which hGH can influence.

hGH is produced by the somatotroph cells of the anterior pituitary and its secretion is promoted by the hormone somatocrinin and inhibited by the hormone somatostatin, both of which are produced by the hypothalamus. hGH has direct effects (via membrane receptors) on lipolysis (increase) and on glucose metabolism (reduction), both of these effects occurring synergistically with cortisol. The effects of hGH on growth are indirect, that is hGH releases 'growth promoting factors', known collectively as the somatomedins, from the liver and possibly from other tissues as well. These growth factors, principally somatomedin A and somatomedin C (which is also called IGF1) mediate many of the growth stimulating aspects of hGH. The principal growth effect of interest to athletes is skeletal growth. Somatomedin C increases cartilage production in the long bones mainly at the epiphyses. Each long bone has, at each end, an epiphysis or epiphyseal plate consisting of a thin disc of cartilage, situated a short distance from the head of the bone. The cartilage cells or chondrocytes multiply following stimulation by somatomedin C which appears to increase directly the synthesis of the polysaccharide constituent of cartilage, chandroitin sulphate. Cartilage production (and its subsequent conversion to mature bone) occurs throughout infancy reaching a peak during the pubertal 'growth sport'. Cartilage deposition is eventually terminated and bone growth arrested probably by the increasing plasma level of sex hormones during later adolescence. Thus, as cartilage deposition ceases the epiphyseal plate becomes completely converted to bone and epiphyseal closure is said to have occurred. Once this stage has been reached no further bone elongation can occur.

hGH has been used legitimately for over 40 years for the treatment of hGH dependent growth disorders. Thus, ateliotic dwarfs, whose deficient growth is due to insufficient hGH secretion can be treated with hGH and assume a normal adult range for their race. However, the treatment with hGH must be completed before adolescence, that is before epiphyseal closure has begun. Until recently, hGH was in short supply because its only source was the pituitary glands obtained at autopsy from dead humans. Synthetic hGH will, however, soon be available to treat human dwarfism and also, unfortunately, for abuse by athletes.

It has been realized for some time that 'cosmetic' increases in height could be induced in normally growing children by treating them with hGH, for example to ensure that they grew tall enough to qualify for the police, marines or ballet school. Such treatment was quite unethical since it drew on the scarce supplies of the hormone needed to treat genuine patients. How easy it would be, then, to produce taller athletes who would be at a particular advantage in jumping and vaulting events and in sports such as basketball. Taylor (1985) has described the increasing temptation to give hGH to pre-pubertal childen of athletic promise in order to produce a group of super athletic giants. Tallness is not always an advantage in sport, for example in gymnastics, but most importantly, with hGH administration comes the risk of serious side effects in later life. The major side effect of excessive hGH adminis-tration is the group of symptoms which give rise to the condition known as acromegaly. This condition includes hyperglycaemia, enlarged internal organs, thickening and coarsening of the skin, lack of subcutaneous fat, coarsening of facial features including overgrowth of the lower jaw, and orbital bones and enlargement of the tongue. The fingers and toes increase in length and an extreme form of osteoarthritis may occur. This condition is normally caused by a tumour of the pituitary somatotroph cells causing hypersecretion of hGH. Taylor (1985) has described several cases of acromegaly in athletes who have taken hGH, including one whose skin was so thickened that it would resist the penetration of a hypodermic needle!

Given these dangerous side effects why abuse hGH? The simple answer is that hGH unlike anabolic steroids increases stature while simultaneously inducing some increase in muscle size. Most important of all, hGH abuse is at present undetectable because synthetic hGH is identical with the endogenous hormone and the two cannot, at present, be distinguished from one another. Also, hGH abuse will have occurred before adolescence so that any evidence of injection will be absent in the adult and the appalling side effects will probably only emerge insidiously in early middle age when most athletes have retired from national and international competitions.

2.6 Postscript – Seoul 1988

By the end of the Seoul Olympics, ten competitors had been found to have prohibited substances in their urine. While the British sprinter, Linford Christie, was acquitted, the 100 metres champion, Ben Johnson, spectacularly failed to satisfy the IOC medical committee about the presence of the anabolic steroid stanozolol or its metabolites in his urine. Johnson's gold medal was withdrawn despite his coach's protests that a post-event drink may have been 'spiked' with the drug.

Despite its popularity, stanozolol is a strange choice for transgressors. Though possessing the same basic chemical ring structure as other anabolic steroids it has, in its structure, an additional 1,2 diazole ring containing two nitrogen atoms. There is no way that this compound could be confused with any other chemical compound in drug tests, except perhaps danozol which is also an anabolic steroid. Of all the anabolics, stanozolol is uniquely resistant to metabolism, possessing, in addition to the biochemically stable diazole ring, a 17α-methyl group (Figure 2.1). Thus stanozolol administration will lead to a series of unusual and unique metabolites.

The use of 2–3 month drug holidays in order to elude the dope detectors is also dubious. Pharmacokinetics, the study of how the body handles drugs, can predict how long a drug will remain in the blood or over what period it will be excreted in the urine. However, some steroid drugs have notoriously complex routes of metabolism in that they may, on reaching the liver, be secreted into the bile, released back into the small intestine and be reabsorbed from the large intestine, thus prolonging their retention by the plasma and the whole body. There are also very marked inter-individual and inter-racial variations in the rate at which steroid drugs are metabolized and so someone who inactivates and eliminates the drug at a slower than average rate can expect to retain the drug for longer. Administration of anabolic steroids also suppresses natural testosterone secretion (page 73) and so an abnormally low plasma testosterone level is additionally indicative of anabolic steroid-taking. While identifying Johnson as the 'loser', the press have failed to name the real winners of this Olympic contest: a team gold should go to the scientists and technicians of the Korean Advanced Institute of Science and Technology and their coach, Professor Jong-Sei Park.

2.7 References

Costill, D. L., Pearson, D. R. and Fink, W. J. (1984) Anabolic steroid use among athletes. Changes in HDL-C levels. *Physician and Sports Medicine*, **12**, 113–17.

Freed, D. L. J., Banks, A. J., Longson, D. and Burley, D. M. (1975) Anabolic steroids in athletics: cross-over double blind trial in weightlifters. *Br. Med. J.*, **2**, 471–3.

Goldman, B. (1984) *Death in the Locker Room: steroids and sports.* Century Publishing, London.

Hervey, G. R. (1982) What are the effects of anabolic steroids? In *Science and Sporting Performance: Management or Manipulation?* (eds B. Davies and G. Thomas), Oxford University Press, Oxford, pp. 121–36.

Hervey, G. R., Knibbs, A. V., Burkinshaw, L., Morgan, D. B., Jones, P. R. M., Chettle, D. R. and Vartsky, D. (1981) Effects of methandione on the performance and body composition of man undergoing athletic training. *Clin. Sci.*, **60**, 457–61.

Holma, P. K. (1979) Effects of an anabolic steroid (methandienone) on spermatogenesis. *Contraception*, **15**, 151–62.

Ryan, A. J. (1981) Anabolic steroids are fool's gold. *Fedn. Proc.*, **40**, 2682–8.

Tanner, J. (1962) *Growth at Adolescence.* Blackwell Scientific Publications, Oxford.

Taylor, W. N. (1985) *Hormonal Manipulation.* Macfarland, London.

Wright, J. E. (1980) Anabolic steroids and athletics. *Exercise and Sport Science Research*, **8**, 149–202.

3 Drug treatment of inflammation in sports injuries

P. N. C. ELLIOTT

3.1 Summary

Following a brief introduction putting sports injury in perspective, the nature of the inflammatory response is described. The role of chemical mediators of inflammation and the contribution of leucocytes to the inflammation is detailed.

The treatment of sporting injuries is then discussed with particular reference to the use of aerosol sprays, aspirin-like drugs, proteolytic enzymes and anti-inflammatory glucocorticoids. The place of each therapy is discussed and possible mechanisms of action of the drugs outlined.

3.2 Introduction

All sports have developed from the natural capabilities of the human mind and body and so, when partaken at a modest level, few sports involve great risk of physical injury. This situation changes, however, when sporting pursuits are undertaken at higher competitive levels. As it becomes necessary to push the body further, in an effort to achieve greater performance, a point may well be reached where the stresses and strains exerted on the structural framework of the body may exceed that which the body is capable of withstanding, resulting in connective tissues being torn and joints being dislocated. Many sports carry their own peculiar additional risks of injury to the body; the boxer may suffer repeated blows to the face causing extensive bruising and laceration and the footballer may receive kicks to the legs resulting in bruising or even bone fracture.

Any traumatic injury to a sportsman will result in a reduced level of performance capability and may require abstention from sport for a period of recuperation. As well as the pain and personal discomfort associated with injury the person's performance is unlikely to be improved during a period of inactivity and may indeed require an extended subsequent training period to regain peak fitness.

In a sport where a career may be of limited duration and where there is a short season of competition the result of even minor trauma may be devastating. To the keen amateur, years of training may be wasted by an inability to participate competitively in a once in a lifetime event; to the top international professional a day on the bench may represent the loss of vast sums of money to the individual or their club. Whatever the injury one of its undoubted features will be the occurrence of an inflammatory reaction at the damaged site.

3.3 The inflammatory response

Inflammation (from the Latin inflammare, meaning to set on fire) is a term widely employed to describe the pathological process which occurs at the site of tissue damage. A precise definition of the condition is difficult. In 1890 it was defined as 'the reaction of irritated and damaged tissues which still retain vitality', whilst more recently it has been argued that this description is too restricted and that 'inflammation is a process which begins following a sub-lethal injury to tissues and ends with complete healing' would be a better definition. Neither of these definitions indicate the underlying nature of the process so, perhaps, a more definitive description would be that it is a process which enables the concentration of the body's defensive and regenerative resources into an area of challenge or damage. Undoubtedly the classical description of the signs of inflammation was given by Celcus in the first century AD, in his De re medicinia: 'indeed the signs of inflammation are four, redness and swelling with heat and pain'. To these four signs was added a fifth – loss of function – by Virchow (1858) the founder of modern cellular pathology.

Inflammation is a process which is fundamentally important for survival. Protection against noxious stimuli and the repair of damaged tissue are essential processes. That inflammation is merely a defensive process, however, has been challenged. It has been proposed that without an inflammatory response organisms would tend to form symbiotic relationships with a resultant loss of individual identity. This tendency for organisms to incorporate each other into a single system would inhibit biological diversity. Thus without inflammation no evolution could occur!

Even before the start of the 20th century the processes of inflammation were studied, the principal tool employed at that time being the microscope. Defense mechanisms typical of those seen in mammals were found in many lower organisms. At that time it was maintained that the primary movement of the inflammatory reaction was the direction of protoplasm to digest any noxious agent. This activity can be seen in many different phyla of the animal kingdom. In protozoans, phagocytic (that is engulfing) activity is exerted by the organism as a whole, but in higher animals this function is attributed to specialized cells. The phagocytic cells of multicellular organisms are able to move to the site of the noxious agent by amoeboid movement. This movement is greatly enhanced in, but not restricted to, those organisms having a vascular system for transport of these cells to the affected area. If the reaction of primitive organisms to noxious stimuli can be termed inflammation, then it is clear that the classical signs of the reaction will not be seen in inflammation of lower animals. Without a vascular system there can be no redness or heat, and indeed with the exception of mammals and birds which are warm-blooded, inflammation of the tissues of animal species will not be accompanied by heat at the affected site.

Some 19th century physiologists also recognized the importance of the circulation and proposed that it was the vascular system itself that was responsible for inflammation. Undoubtedly the vascular system is of fundamental importance in the inflammatory process of mammals but it is as well to remember that the evolutionary forerunner of this process may not have been a vascular reaction.

However inflammation may be defined, it is a dynamic process and this process may on occasions be capable of causing more harm to the organism than the initiating noxious stimulus. For example, the necrotic lesions produced on dogs at the site of feeding of the tick can be virtually eliminated by the prior destruction of polymorphs. Similarly, in some immunologically induced reactions considerable tissue damage can result from sensitivity to seemingly harmless agents. There is no obvious reason why the inflammatory reactions such as rheumatic fever or rheumatoid arthritis benefit an organism. Clearly not all inflammation can be useful. The combined effect of the components of the body's defensive mechanism may often be excessive.

Whilst there are many and varied kinds of inflammation (and of the many factors which can be involved some may be lacking or unimportant in certain inflammations) it is possible to consider that the basic components of the inflammatory reaction may be due to the combined effects of changes in the microcirculation, alteration of permeability of the vessel walls and emigration of leucocytes, chemotaxis and phagocytosis.

3.3.1 CHANGES IN THE MICROCIRCULATION DURING THE INFLAMMATORY RESPONSE

The immediate reaction of skin to a burn or irritant is to become red. This reddening will persist for a variable time depending on the severity of the stimulus. The redness is due to an increased volume of blood flowing through the inflamed area. Consequently the temperature of the inflamed skin rises and approaches that of the deep body temperature. This effect on the microcirculation is seen clearly if a firm line is drawn with a blunt point over a surface of the forearm. As Lewis demonstrated in 1927, a red line appears in exactly the position that the stimulus was applied. This dull red area is then surrounded by a bright red halo and a weal begins to form firstly at the red line and then spreading outwards. Lewis confirmed earlier suggestions that many different types of injury, besides mechanical injury, could induce inflammation including heat, cold, electric shock, radiation and chemical irritants.

Detailed study of vascular changes occurring during inflammation has been made by many physiologists by observing over long periods vascular changes in sheets of connective tissue arranged on a microscope stage. In this way it has been demonstrated that the whole capillary bed at the damaged site becomes suffused with blood at an increased pressure. Capillaries dilate and many closed ones open up. The venules dilate and there is an increased flow of blood in the draining veins. This rapid flow gradually slows in the central capillaries and venules even though the vessels are still dilated. This slowing may gradually spread to the peripheral areas of the lesion and the flow may even stop completely. Despite this stasis the capillary pressure remains high probably due to a resistance to outflow. The pressure in the small veins may be increased by a rise in pressure of the interstitial fluid due to oedema. Two of the cardinal signs of inflammation – heat and redness – are caused by this increase in blood flow to the affected area. A third cardinal sign – swelling – is also due to a change in the vascular system. In this case it is a change in the permeability of the blood vessel wall to protein. Normally the fluid found outside the blood system, in the tissues, is composed of water with some low molecular weight solutes such as sodium chloride; the protein content of this fluid is very low. However, the protein content of blood is relatively high and this state of affairs is maintained by virtue of the fact that the blood vessel wall is permeable only to water and salts. Water is forced out of small blood vessels at the arteriolar end of capillary beds due to the internal pressure which is generated by the heart on the enclosed vascular system. Without the colloid osmotic pressure exerted by the plasma protein causing this water to be drawn back into the blood system, blood volume would very rapidly diminish due to the net movement of water from the blood to the tissues. At the inflammatory site the permeability of small blood vessels changes to allow plasma protein to leak out of the vessel into the surrounding tissue and this change in distribution of protein is followed by a net passage of water from the blood into the tissues giving rise to the oedema which may ultimately be seen as a swelling. Electron microscopic examination of blood vessels to which vasoactive substances were applied revealed the production of gaps 0.1–0.4 μm in diameter between adjacent endothelial cells. These gaps were found to be temporary and there was no apparent damage caused to the endothelium of the leaking vessel.

Even though all inflammatory reactions are unique, very similar reactions can be induced by widely differing stimuli. This has led to the idea that some intermediary system exists between the stimulus and the effect which links them together. The most popular idea is that the inflammatory insult causes the release of chemicals within the body which then trigger the inflammatory reactions. This mediator concept was exemplified by Lewis (1927) who proposed that the local vasodilatation and increased vascular permeability observed in the triple response could be mediated by a substance, liberated by the tissue, which he termed H-substance. The search for chemical mediators of inflammation has been particularly directed towards finding substances capable of increasing vascular permeability, largely because this parameter may be quantified quite easily. It should be remembered, however, that mediators of increased vascular permeability may not necessarily be responsible for mediation of other aspects of the inflammatory reaction. The time course of vasodilatation and increased vascular permeability differ markedly from each other in many types of inflammatory reactions induced by chemical irritants. Investigation of the mediation of permeability changes in general concerns endogenous substances; these can be demonstrated in normal or inflamed tissue which have high permeability increasing potency. A number of such substances have been investigated to determine their possible role in the inflammatory response.

One of the first substances examined as a potential mediator of inflammation was histamine. Histamine is formed by the decarboxylation of the amino acid histidine and is a normal constituent of most tissues. The most abundant source of histamine in the body is to be found in the mast cells where it is stored in granules in association with the anti-coagulant substance heparin. Mast cells are found in high levels in the lungs, gastrointestinal system and skin. When released from the mast cell, or when injected, histamine produces vasodilatation and an increase in blood vessel permeability. At high concentrations histamine can also induce pain and so this particular locally acting hormone has the properties that could contribute to all four cardinal signs of inflammation.

Histamine has been found to be released following chemical, thermal and immunological challenge and after ionizing irradiation. The contribution of histamine to most inflammatory reactions is limited, however, to the very early phase and in most cases after a few hours antihistamine drugs have no anti-inflammatory activity. The most notable exception is in the case of immunological reactions where histamine activity may persist throughout the duration of a type I hypersensitivity reaction such as hay fever or urticaria (Figure 3.1), where anti-histamine drugs represent an effective therapeutic approach.

The body can generate a number of highly active polypeptide hormones which exert local actions on the tissues in a variety of circumstances. A characteristic feature of these substances is that they are intensely vaso-active. One particular group of these polypeptides are known as the kinins and the best known of these is bradykinin – a polypeptide of nine amino acid residues. Kinins can be released in all body fluids by the action of an enzyme, kallikrein, on a globulin protein. In glandular tissue, kinins may be responsible for the functional vasodilatation that occurs during periods of glandular activity. During

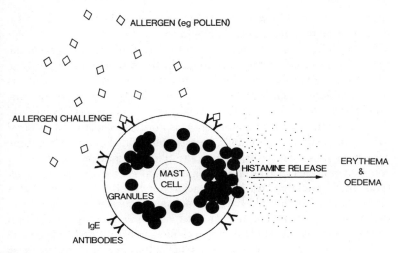

Figure 3.1 Histamine release in allergic reactions.

exercise, bradykinin may be released in response to the increasing acidity that occurs in active muscles and causes vasodilatation of the tissues and promotes sweating. It is possible that kinins may contribute to ischaemic pain where the vasodilatation has proved inadequate. Kinins are also generated where tissue damage occurs and may promote both vasodilatation and an increase in blood vessel permeability. They are extremely potent in these respects but are very labile, having a half-life in blood of only a few seconds. Despite the difficulties that exist in handling the material, some evidence has been produced indicating that kinins do contribute to inflammatory reactions but, as with histamine, this may well be restricted to the fairly early stages of an acute reaction.

A substance capable of inhibiting kallikrein has been detected in a number of bovine tissues. This substance, aprotinin, is available commercially and has been tried in the treatment of acute pancreatitis where it owes its possible usefulness to inhibiting the release of kinins and to blocking the activity of pancreatic proteases. It has been shown to be active as an anti-inflammatory agent in experimental animals but clinical trials in human inflammatory diseases have failed to provide convincing evidence of efficacy. It would seem, therefore, that whilst kinins may contribute to the early development of an inflammatory reaction their inhibition would not seem to be an important target for drug treatment in musculoskeletal injuries.

Perhaps the most significant area of interest, in recent years, in the mediation of inflammatory reaction is in the products of arachidonic acid. Every cell in the body has the capacity to generate some products from arachidonic acid which is a 20 carbon straight chain polyunsaturated fatty acid. This substance is usually found only at very low levels in the free form, but an abundant supply is normally available in a bound form, principally as cell membrane phospholipid. Following hormone activity or perturbation of the cell the phospholipids are split by the action of enzymes such as phospholipase A_2 to release arachidonic acid. Once made available, arachidonic acid is metabolized in a way that is characteristic for the cell. This metabolism is generally rapid since it is the availability of arachidonic acid that is the rate limiting factor. Two enzyme systems are available for this metabolism: a cyclo-oxygenase and a lipoxygenase. None of the biologically active products of these enzymes have long half-lives in the body and they are not generally stored. They tend to exert their activities locally and it has become apparent that many of them have properties which conflict with each other giving rise to the idea that they are involved in the local modulation of physiological processes.

The first class of these products to be discovered was the prostaglandins, so named because it was thought that they were secreted by the prostate gland although it was subsequently found that the principal source of these substances found in seminal fluid was the seminal vesicles. Prostaglandins are formed by the action of cyclo-oxygenase on arachidonic acid. This enzyme causes the oxygenation and internal cyclization of the fatty acid to give an unstable cyclic endoperoxide PGG_2. This unstable 15-hydroperoxy compound rapidly reduces to the 15-hydroxy derivative PGH_2 this change being accompanied by the release of a free radical into the medium. It is worthy of mention here that free radicals are extremely damaging to biological tissues and may be responsible for some of the tissue destruction that occurs in the course of inflammatory reactions. The second stage of synthesis involves another enzyme which is tissue specific and results in the conversion of the cyclic endoperoxide to either PGE_2, $PGF_{2\alpha}$, PGI or to a thromboxane depending on the tissue (Figure 3.2).

Tremendous interest has been shown in these highly biologically-active substances since the discovery of their presence in exudates. A number of properties exhibited by prostaglandins are compatible with

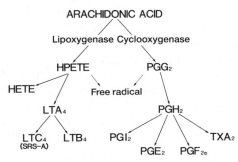

Figure 3.2 Some biologically active metabolites of arachidonic acid.

the idea that these locally acting hormones are mediators of the inflammatory response. Firstly, they can cause profound vasodilatation at a very low concentration and the erythema that they induce is very long lasting, persisting even after the prostaglandins have been broken down. Prostaglandins by themselves do not greatly affect vascular permeability nor do they evoke a pain response at physiological concentration. Prostaglandins do, however, radically exaggerate the vascular permeability-increasing and pain-reducing activity of other substances such as histamine and bradykinin. These properties, coupled with the fact that raised prostaglandin levels are readily detectable in a number of inflammatory conditions, make them ideal candidates for the role of mediators of inflammation.

3.3.2 LEUCOCYTES IN INFLAMMATION

Some types of inflammatory reaction such as acute allergic responses are restricted to changes in the microcirculation alone. More chronic conditions of the type common to sports injuries involve another major physiological change, that is the influx of leucocytes.

Normal tissues contain few extravascular polymorphs but in an inflammatory reaction these cells may pass from the microcirculation into the damaged tissue site. Following an injury, blood polymorphs stick momentarily to the endothelium; they roll along the inside surface of the vessel wall, adhering briefly until they re-enter the circulation. After a few minutes, more and more cells adhere and eventually these are not dislodged by the blood flow. In this way the endothelium comes to be lined. This process is called margination. Other leucocytes, platelets, and red cells may also stick. The marginated polymorphs leave the intravascular site by emigrating or diapedesis. A pseudopodium insinuates itself between the endothelial cells and the bulk of the polymorph, including the nucleus, passes between the endothelial cells and comes to lie outside the endothelial cell but within the basement membrane. The manner in which the cell passes through the basement membrane is not known. These cells make an important contribution to the inflammatory process; this has been demonstrated by the reduced inflammatory response that occurs in experimental animals when their polymorphonuclear leucocytes have been depleted. To achieve this reduction, the number of circulating polymorphs and polymorphs which enter the circulation (presumably from the bone marrow) following an inflammatory stimulus must be reduced to very low levels.

Polymorphonuclear leucocytes are the first circulating cells to accumulate in large numbers in an injured area. These cells are phagocytic and play a protective role by ingesting and subsequently digesting invading micro-organisms or tissue debris in the affected area. Polymorphs do not survive for more than a few hours outside the circulation and when they die they release their contents, which include a wide range of catabolic enzymes, into the surrounding area resulting in further damage to the tissues.

As well as the emigration of polymorphonuclear cells from the blood there is also a movement of mononuclear cells. Monocytes begin to move into the affected site at the same time as the polymorphs but they are slower and are therefore generally outnumbered by polymorphonuclear cells at the start of a reaction. Mononuclear cells are, however, much more enduring than the polymorphs and in many reactions begin to predominate after a day or so. Outside the circulation, monocytes go through a maturation phase becoming macrophages which, as the name implies, are large phagocytic cells. These cells can undergo cell division which also contributes to the large number of mononuclear cells which accumulate at the inflamed site.

In the same way that changes in the microcirculation are brought about by chemical mediation the influx of leucocytes is also subject to chemical control. The simplest explanation for the phenomenon of cell migration is that a chemical stimulus originating from the damaged site is recognized by leucocytes which respond by moving along a concentration gradient of the chemical towards the highest concentration; this process is called chemotaxis. There are a number of chemotactic substances known to be released from inflammatory sites and whilst cells may respond in a minor way to the mediators which effect changes in the vasculature the most potent agents have little effect on the microcirculation.

Arachidonic acid can be metabolized by a lipoxygenase system to generate a range of hydroxyeicosatetraenoic acids one of which is 5,12 dihydroxyeicosatetraenoic acid or leucotriene B_4(LTB$_4$). LTB$_4$ is a potent chemotactic agent for polymorphonuclear leucocytes and mononuclear cells. LTB$_4$ also stimulates the general activity of leucocytes as well as inducing more rapid movement and the release of degradative enzymes into the area. Thus, when arachidonic acid is released from cell membranes the resultant prostaglandins and leucotrienes produced may, between them, mediate the development of all the major processes involved in an inflammatory response.

Another important source of chemotactic agents is the complement system. This is a complex system of plasma proteins which can be activated by a variety of stimuli including antigen–antibody interaction and endotoxin release to produce a powerful cytolytic, membrane-attack unit. In the course of this activation a number of fragments of the complement components, which are powerfully chemotactic, are released into the area. These include components $C3_a$ and $C5_a$, which are also potent histamine releasers, and the aggregate C567 fraction. The complement system represents about 10% of plasma protein and has been implicated in a variety of inflammatory reactions. Other chemotactic material can be released from the breakdown of the structural protein collagen and from the breakdown of the blood-clotting protein fibrin.

The contributions of the leucocytes to the inflammatory reactions are various. The presence of cells capable of phagocytosis at an injured site is an advantage. The removal of damaged tissues and any foreign material such as micro-organisms is of obvious importance. The local increase in leucocyte numbers at the site of inflammation at least warrants the hypothesis that there is a general increase in the concentration of proteolytic enzymes, because the lysosomes of the leucocytes contain cathepsins and hydrolases and the mast cells are rich in proteolytic enzymes. Release of these enzymes may be an important factor in the maintenance of inflammation by the production of altered tissue proteins and by the non-specific activation of thrombin, kinin forming and plasmin systems. Polymorphs also provide a source of enzymes with more specific activities for maintaining the inflammatory reaction. The release of kininogenases from polymorphs has been reported, and the presence of a specific collagenase in human polymorphs has been noted. In some experimental models of inflammation, the phase in which prostaglandins are released corresponds in time to the migration of leucocytes into the inflamed area, and it has been proposed that the main source of prostaglandins at the inflammatory site are the polymorphs.

The initial reaction to most types of injury is an acute inflammatory response exhibiting the prominent feature of increased vascular permeability. This reaction will normally resolve in time, and if actual tissue necrosis is slight no identifiable trace of the reaction will be left. In a more severe situation, repair is effected by the synthesis of connective tissue to form a scar.

In some circumstances, however, inflammation may persist. This chronic reaction may be caused by the presence of some foreign material which is not easily removed from the inflammatory site. It has been found that the resolution of an inflammatory lesion is invariably associated with the disappearance of the inflammatory inducing irritant, but persistent inflammation may not necessarily be caused by any detectable irritant – for example the aetiology of rheumatoid arthritis is uncertain. The characteristic feature of chronic inflammation is the presence of white cells at the site of reaction. Some acute inflammatory reactions, such as the dextran-induced paw oedema in the rat, may proceed without migration of white cells into the extravascular spaces of the paw, but chronic inflammation is invariably associated with large numbers of extravascular white cells. Chronic inflammation is characterized by concurrent tissue destruction and resultant inflammation. The death of invading polymorphs at an inflamed site with the resultant release of all the cellular enzymes can give rise to a suppurative lesion. A suppurative lesion may continue at the site of some foreign material but the necrotic area may become surrounded by a deposition of fibrous material and white cells to give rise to an abscess. A separation of degenerative and synthetic processes as in the case of an abscess is not always seen, the two processes often occurring simultaneously at the same site. Such a chronic inflammatory mass is called a granuloma.

Chronic inflammation can occur, however, without passing through an acute or suppurative phase by the gradual development directly into the chronic state. Histological examination of chronic inflammatory lesions reveals the presence of a variety of different types of white cell. In rheumatoid synovial fluids large numbers of white cells, principally polymorphs, can be found. These have extremely short half-lives of the order of only 3–4 hours and the variety of damaging agents which can be released from these cells has already been outlined. Polymorphs are also actively phagocytic but this function may not be important in chronic inflammatory situations since their short life span will frequently result in the release of any ingested material on the death of the cell. The predominant variety of polymorph is the neutrophil, but eosinophilic polymorphs, which share many of the properties of the neutrophil, also occur in inflammatory foci, possibly as a marker of general polymorph involvement although in certain reactions the eosinophilic polymorph may predominate.

Most chronic inflammatory reactions are characterized by the presence of large numbers of mononuclear cells. Those mononuclear cells in a chronic inflammatory state may be derived either by immigration or by division and the persistence of these cells may be due to their great longevity. Macrophages, like polymorphs, are phagocytic and their ability to engulf appears to be important since the removal of foreign material and tissue debris is necessary for resolution of a reaction.

Within an area of chronic inflammation macrophages may be transformed into two other cell types: epitheloid cells and foreign body giant cells. Epitheloid cells are a common feature of granulomatous inflammation and can be produced by natural maturation of macrophages if they live long enough; they do not have undigested phagocytosed material within the cell. Giant cells are multinucleate and have been shown to be produced by cell fusion although this fusion may be followed by nuclear division without cytoplasmic fission. These cells are found in large numbers around foreign bodies which are too large for macrophages to engulf. Other cells present in chronic inflammatory reactions are fibroblasts, which are probably derived from local connective tissue fibroblasts and are responsible for collagen deposition, and lymphocytes and plasma cells which are responsible for the production of antibodies which facilitate the elimination of microorganisms.

The contribution that any of the factors examined here may make in the inflammatory sequelae to a sporting injury cannot be specified but undoubtedly there will be: an increased influx of blood giving rise to the characteristic heat and redness, a movement of plasma protein and associated water into the tissue, causing swelling and pain due, perhaps, to pressure on the nerve endings caused by the swelling or to the effect of released chemical mediators of pain, and finally, and perhaps most importantly to the sportsman, there will be loss of function – Virchow's fifth cardinal sign. The persistence of the problem depends on many factors but certainly the influx of leucocytes and the release of their enzyme-rich contents will compound the damage already caused and tend to prolong the duration of the reaction. Given that no further aggravation occurs and that there are no complications, resolution should occur within days or weeks and at worst months. A pertinent question to ask at this point is whether the inflammation that follows a traumatic injury is necessary. Clearly the body automatically takes the safest course of action when injured and directs its defense systems to the area to make sure that no microbial invasion occurs and that all the necessary resources are made available to repair the damage. It is evident, however, that the body has a tendency to over-react. The response in many cases may be more serious than the stimulus.

3.4 The treatment of sporting injuries

A number of treatments are available to deal with sporting injuries by the reduction of pain and inflammation. It is clear, however, that great care must be taken in judging the severity of an injury. Pain is the cue that intimates the severity of a problem. There are many drugs which can reduce our appreciation of pain, but a reduction of pain sensation may lead to the induction of further damage to an injury due to the failure to respond to the natural inclination to rest. Clear evidence of the dangers of masking pain sensation can be seen amongst those who suffer peripheral mutilation common amongst people with impaired sensory nerve activity such as untreated lepers.

A common sight these days is the arrival on the field of play of the trainer who reaches into his bag for the aerosol can with which he sprays some area of the prostrated sportsman he is attending. The injured player stands gingerly, and, cautiously at first, he runs on, the trainer collects up his bag with his 'magic' spray and walks off. These aerosol sprays contain volatile compounds which evaporate on the skin surface causing rapid chilling of the area. The practice of cooling an injured area by volatile spray, cold compress or ice-pack, if applied rapidly, may well reduce the immediate response to minor trauma by inhibiting the active processes which are involved in the initiation of an inflammatory reaction. Problems have arisen because of the abuse of these solvent based products for 'sniffing'. Other topical applications which are used successfully for the treatment of injured tissues include liniments. These preparations are rubefacients and act by counter irritation. This is a phenomenon where mild or moderate pain can be relieved by irritating the skin. Counter irritation is effective in providing relief from painful lesions of muscles, tendons and joints. There is, however, little evidence that the topical application of preparations containing adrenaline or aspirin is of value in the relief of pain.

3.4.1 THE MODES OF ACTION OF ANTI-INFLAMMATORY DRUGS

Although the treatment of inflammation with anti-inflammatory agents was practiced by Hippocrates, who recommended the chewing of willow bark for a variety of ailments, the use of such measures was largely forsaken during subsequent centuries. It was not until 1876 when a physician named Maclagan, who was unimpressed with the treatments that were available for rheumatic fever (a condition characterized by extensive inflammatory lesions) which included such measures as blood letting, revolutionized the treatment of this condition by the reintroduction of an extract of willow bark called salicin. A synthetic analogue of this glycoside was soon produced and in 1899 a German pharmaceutical company, Bayer, introduced a more palatable derivative, acetylsalicylic acid under the trade name Aspirine. Almost 100 years later we still have aspirin readily available as a simple, cheap and effective remedy for a wide variety of ailments. It has been the subject of innumerable clinical trials in many diverse areas of medicine ranging from the treatment of food intolerance to the prevention of heart attacks. Without doubt, though, the bulk of the tens of thousands of tons of aspirin consumed each year is taken for the alleviation of pain, inflammation and fever.

There are now about 20 aspirin-like drugs available for clinical use although only aspirin and ibuprofen are available for general purchase. These aspirin-like drugs all have proven anti-inflammatory activity in the treatment of chronic inflammatory conditions such as rheumatoid arthritis. Countless clinical trials have demonstrated the efficacy of these agents in alleviating both objective and subjective symptoms of inflammatory disease. Whilst some of these agents are more popular than others there is no clear indication that any one drug is more effective than any other. Indeed it is difficult to find convincing proof that any of the new drugs in this class is more effective than aspirin. The assessment of activity of this type of drug is, however, fraught with difficulties. It is not easy to find large numbers of patients with similar disease states who are prepared to be subjected to the withdrawal of active drugs in order to act as controls in such trials, and it is not easy to quantitate a reduction in inflammation. Given that these difficulties exist when testing drugs on common chronic conditions it can be perceived that the difficulties involved in testing anti-inflammatory agents in acute sporting injuries, which may affect any part of the body, are considerably greater. Since a chronically inflamed joint in a patient with rheumatoid arthritis may remain in a similar condition for weeks on end, the effect of introduction and withdrawal of an effective anti-inflammatory agent on the level of inflammation of that joint should be seen fairly easily. Following a traumatic sporting injury, however, it is probable that the inflamed part will progressively heal over a fairly limited period without intervention. How, then, can you measure the efficacy of an anti-inflammatory drug superimposed on a naturally regressing inflammatory condition? The simple answer is: with great difficulty! The majority of clinical trials published on the efficacy of aspirin-like drugs in sports injury are organized with two groups of injured sportsmen, each given a different member of this group of drugs. Usually no significant difference is established between the two drugs under test. Whilst these drugs are clearly effective in the treatment of chronic disease, evidence that they do have a role to play in acute traumatic injury treatment is much more limited. To firmly establish that drugs like aspirin can effectively treat a sports injury a number of criteria would have to be met. Firstly, suitable injuries, preferably all of a certain type, would be needed in reasonble numbers. Secondly, some measure of effectiveness would be required which would have clear meaning. Thirdly, a comparison would have to be made with a group of similar patients receiving no drug treatment, that is a control group. Because many individuals are responsive to suggestion, this control group would have to be given what appears to be the same treatment as the test group but with the active drug missing. In other words one group would be given the drug whilst the other group would be given identical looking tablets but containing no drug, so-called placebos.

Now with regard to the first two criteria perhaps a good place to look for a plentiful supply of similar sports injuries would be in a club where members are involved in the same sport and, therefore, the same injury tendencies. A measurement of the period of time following injury until the injured person is fit for competition or full training again could serve as the key to assess effectiveness. If this time is reduced in the drug-treated group then it could be concluded that the drug was a success. With regard to the third criteria, however, there is a substantial ethical and moral problem. If the drug works or even if it is thought to work, it is difficult to justify the withholding of that treatment for the purpose of a trial since this action might prolong unnecessarily the period of absence from the sport, which in many professional clubs would be an unacceptable action.

Despite the relative paucity of convincing trials which demonstrate the effectiveness of these anti-inflammatory drugs their use in the treatment of sports injuries is very widespread. The commencement of a course of aspirin-like drugs immediately after the injury occurs appears to be an effective way to reduce the recovery time. The most commonly used drugs in this class are aspirin, indomethacin, naproxen, piroxicam and ibuprofen. The use of these drugs, though widespread, remains largely empirical as there is no universally accepted explanation as to how they reduce inflammation. Indeed our understanding of the processes involved in soft tissue injury is far from complete. A number of suggestions have been made however to explain the anti-inflammatory activity of the aspirin-like drugs. Considerable attention has been focused on the possible interaction of these drugs with various factors involved in this inflammatory process. For example, many early attempts to explain the anti-inflammatory activity of these drugs considered their ability to interfere with proteolytic enzymes. These enzymes are involved, both in the early stages of inflammation, and in the later stages when the process is well established. An inhibition of proteolytic enzyme activity either at the start of the reaction, preventing the activation of the complement, kinin, fibrin or plasmin systems, or during the later, autocatabolic stage of inflammation could be the mechanism of action. Certainly many anti-inflammatory drugs have been shown to have some measure of anti-protease activity, but the general correlation between enzyme inhibition and anti-inflammatory activity is not impressive. Aspirin derivatives are known to inhibit a large number of enzyme systems but inhibition is generally seen only at drug concentrations which exceed the normal therapeutic level. Another explanation which has been proposed that is closely related to this idea is that the anti-inflammatory drugs reduce inflammation by preventing the release of enzymes from lysosomes during the more established phase of the reaction. Again, whilst there is some experimental evidence available to support this idea overall it is not a convincing explanation.

With an improved understanding of the mediation of inflammation came the idea that the action of anti-inflammatory drugs might be due to an interference with the activities of one or more of the proposed chemical mediators of inflammation. It was not, however, until 1971 that any major headway was made in this area of our understanding. In a series of three papers published in *Nature*, John Vane and his colleagues outlined a hypothesis that the action of the aspirin-like drugs could be attributed to their ability to suppress the synthesis of prostaglandins. Virtually all the non-steroidal anti-inflammatory drugs have been shown to inhibit the synthesis of prostaglandins and they generally exhibit this property at concentrations which are low enough to be achieved with normal therapeutic doses of the drugs. The predictable consequences of the inhibition of prostaglandin synthesis on an inflammatory process, based on the known pro-inflammatory activities of the prostaglandins easily lead us to the conclusion that this property of the non-steroidal anti-inflammatory drugs provides an explanation for their mechanisms of action. A reduction in the level of prostaglandins at an inflammatory site should result in a reduction in the symptoms of heat and redness since prostaglandins would normally promote an increased blood flow to the area by virtue of their ability to cause profound erythema. A reduction in the pain associated with the reaction could also be anticipated, since in the absence of prostaglandins there would be no state of hyperalgesia. In other words, the tissues would not exhibit a greater than normal sensitivity to painful stimuli. Oedema would also be reduced in severity as the permeability-increasing effect of chemical agents on blood vessel walls would not be subject to the normal exaggerating action of the prostaglandins. Thus, we can see that the reduction in synthesis of the prostaglandins that can be demonstrated when using the non-steroidal anti-inflammatory drugs could account for the reduction of all the cardinal signs of inflammation. As additional support for this idea of a single, common mechanism of action for the non-steroidal anti-inflammatory drugs, other properties exhibited by this group of drugs can also be explained by an inhibition of prostaglandin synthesis. For example, as well as being analgesic, anti-inflammatory drugs are invariably anti-pyretic agents as well, that is they have the ability to reduce elevated body temperature. Prostaglandins are detectable in increased quantities in the cerebrospinal fluid which fills the cavities of the brain during fever, and it has been shown in animals that the injection of prostaglandins into the anterior hypothalamus evokes a pyrexic response. The inhibition of prostaglandin synthesis, therefore, offers an explanation for this property of these drugs, in addition to their anti-inflammatory action.

Another property which is common to most of these agents is that they inhibit platelet aggregation. To repair damaged blood vessels, platelets come together to form a plug to fill the gap and prevent bleeding. This activity is in part mediated via the synthesis of thromboxanes by the platelets. Drugs such as aspirin which inhibit the cyclo-oxygenase enzyme will prevent the synthesis, not only of prostaglandins but of thromboxanes as well, preventing normal platelet function. In some circumstances, notably when there is already some impairment to normal platelet function, this activity of these drugs may represent a hazard. There is, however, much interest in the potential use of this anti-platelet activity to prevent the development of thrombosis. Small blood clot fragments may lodge in the vascular beds of the brain or heart and it is possible that a very small regular dose of aspirin may protect a subject from a stroke or a heart attack. Another common feature of these agents is their tendency to cause gastric irritation and this, too, can be explained by a mechanism of prostaglandin synthesis inhibition. Prostaglandins normally limit the amount of hydrochloric acid secreted by the parietal cells in the main gastric glands probably by action on the enzyme adenylate cyclase. In addition, prostaglandins may promote the functional vasodilatation necessary for the parietal cells in their secretory mode. If the levels of prostaglandins in the stomach are reduced then a greater amount of acid will be secreted and this acid will be produced by cells which have been forced into this synthetic activity without the usual increased provision of oxygen. This situation may result in gastritis in which some mucosal tissue may be damaged by the ischaemia which can result from the increased metabolic activity without increased blood flow.

Therefore, we have a mechanism of action for the non-steroidal anti-inflammatory drugs which can be invoked to explain, not only their anti-inflammatory activity but also their anti-pyretic and anti-platelet activities, and even serves to explain their most common side effect. This brief account of mechanism would be less than complete, however, if it did not at least indicate one or two of the many observations that have been reported which do not easily fit within this explanation. Firstly, as was made clear in Vane's original paper, sodium salicylate is of the order of 100 times less effective as an inhibitor of prostaglandin synthesis than is acetylsalicylic acid, aspirin, whereas their anti-inflammatory activity is similar. Secondly, in experiments in which inflammation has been induced in animals rendered incapable of generating prostaglandins (by being fed diets deficient in poly-unsaturated fatty acids, e.g. arachidonic acid), aspirin has been shown to be as effective as it is in normal animals. Finally, it has been shown that even small sub-anti-inflammatory doses of aspirin render the inflamed synovial tissue of arthritic joints incapable of producing prostaglandins for several days. Clearly, if this is the mechanism of action of aspirin an explanation is required as to why regular high doses of the drug are needed to achieve an anti-inflammatory action when two or three tablets, two or three times a week would seem to be all that is necessary to induce effective inhibition of prostaglandin synthesis.

The relationship between prostaglandin synthesis and the aspirin-like drugs is, thus, confused. On the one hand, we have a convincing and attractive hypothesis which explains the many and varied activities and even side effects of this group of drugs by one, simple and elegant mechanism. On the other hand, we have evidence that not all anti-inflammatory drugs are good inhibitors of prostaglandin synthesis, that aspirin can exert an anti-inflammatory effect in the absence of any prostaglandin synthesis and that, if anything, it is too good at inhibiting synthesis in rheumatic patients to explain why such large amounts of the drug are needed in clinical practice.

3.4.2 NON-STEROIDAL ANTI-INFLAMMATORY DRUGS IN SPORTS INJURY

Whatever the mechanism by which these drugs exert their effect, their use in the treatment of chronic inflammatory disease is well established and their efficacy beyond question. Similarly, in the treatment of acute traumatic injury their use has become commonplace and although far too many clinical trials have failed to furnish proof of their efficacy, clear evidence that these drugs are of benefit in sports injury has been produced. These drugs represent a simple and safe means of reducing the response to an injury and speeding the return of an injured sportsperson to competitive fitness. Whilst many trials compare the use of two different anti-inflammatory drugs frequently no significant difference between the two drugs is found and where differences are reported they are not consistent. It would, therefore, be difficult to indicate a rank order of efficacy for these drugs. Instead it is proposed to describe the use of some of the commonly used members of this group of drugs in sports injuries. Sprains (rupture of ligaments, which may be

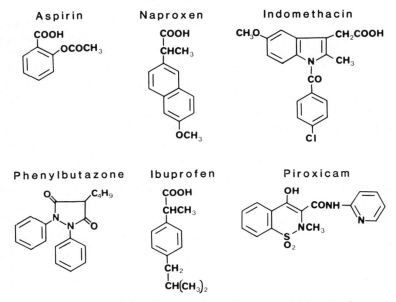

Figure 3.3 Some examples of commonly used non-steroidal anti-inflammatory drugs.

partial), strains (partial tearing of muscles) and bruises are all painful examples of sports injuries. Commonly they may warrant the use of painkilling (analgesic) drugs such as paracetamol or even in severe cases a narcotic analgesic compound such as dihydrocodeine. However, since these conditions are generally associated with an inflammatory component the use of an analgesic drug with anti-inflammatory activity would seem to be a more logical choice. Some examples of common anti-inflammatory drugs are shown in Figure 3.3.

Aspirin

Aspirin is a very effective analgesic drug at a dose of 2–3 g per day. At higher doses, that is in excess of 4 g per day, aspirin will reduce the swelling of an inflamed joint, a property not shown at the lower, analgesic level. Despite the antiquity of this preparation, unequivocal evidence that any of the newer challengers offers an all-round superior performance is lacking. The general availability and low cost of aspirin make it an ideal candidate for self-treatment following sports injury.

Aspirin is, however, not without toxicity although the risks involved with the use of the drug are probably generally overstated. Given that the injured athlete is an otherwise normal, healthy adult, the major problem likely to be encountered following the use of aspirin (or indeed, for that matter, any of the non-steroidal anti-inflammatory drugs) is gastric irritation which may be experienced as a form of dyspepsia. Attempts to reduce this problem by modifying the tablets in a variety of ways have not been particularly successful as it is now generally recognized that the effect of these drugs on the stomach is due not to the unabsorbed drug being in contact with the gastric mucosa, but to the drug being in the circulation. The most effective way to minimize this problem is to avoid the use of these drugs when the stomach is empty. If the drugs are taken following a meal then any increased acid production that ensues can be utilized in the digestive process rather than being free to attack the lining of the stomach itself. In a recent study in which aspirin was compared with naproxen in patients with sports injuries no significant differences were detected between the two drugs although the dose of aspirin used (2 g per day) was arguably on the low side for an anti-inflammatory action (Andersen and Gotzsche, 1984). What this study did demonstrate, however, was that significantly better results were obtained when the interval between injury and the start of treatment was shorter. This effect is widely appreciated now and is exactly what would be predicted from experimental inflammation studies in animals. In laboratory tests of the type used to screen for anti-inflammatory activity of potential new drugs for the treatment of arthritis it can be clearly shown that aspirin-like drugs can profoundly reduce the development of an inflammatory response to an irritant. The effect of these drugs on the inflammatory response to the same irritant after it is established is marginal.

Clearly, if it is deemed necessary to use an anti-inflammatory drug to treat a sports injury it should be given as early as possible after the damage is sustained.

Naproxen

Naproxen has become one of the mainstays of treatment for chronic inflammatory conditions. Its efficacy and safety record are excellent and it is one of the most frequently prescribed drugs for the treatment of arthritis. Since its introduction in the early 1970s naproxen has been the subject of a large number of trials in the treatment of soft tissue injuries and whilst many of these compare naproxen to other non-steroidal anti-inflammatory drugs and find no difference in activity, several trials have shown naproxen to be better than the other drugs in some respects and naproxen has been shown to be superior to placebo. In view of the popularity of this drug and the generally good reports of its efficacy in the literature, naproxen must rank high amongst the most suitable drugs for the treatment of sporting injuries. The drug is given at a dose of 0.5–1 g per day in two or three divided doses. Initially, a high loading dose of 500 or 750 mg may be given to aid the rapid attainment of suitable plasma levels of the drug (750 μg ml^{-1}). The drug may be taken at meal times to help combat any gastric discomfort, although in the presence of food the drug is absorbed more slowly. More rapid absorption occurs with the use of naproxen sodium.

Ibuprofen

Ibuprofen is another non-steroid anti-inflammatory drug with a similar structure to naproxen. It is the oldest propionic acid derivative anti-inflammatory agent in use and considerable experience has, therefore, been obtained with it. This drug is also one of the few drugs of this class available without prescription. It has a reputation for being well tolerated; it is widely felt that it does not induce the same degree of dyspepsia as many of its rivals. It is possible, however, that much of this reputation is based on early experiences with the drug when it was used at relatively low dose levels. To improve the often disappointing activity of ibuprofen the doses used have been increased and whilst the drug is still generally well tolerated it is certainly not without gastric irritant activity at these higher levels. Trials using ibuprofen at doses as low as 1200 mg per day have been shown to reduce pain and recovery time of soft-tissue sports injuries. Hutson (1986) found no significant difference between the activity of ibuprofen given at doses of 1800 mg or 2400 mg daily amongst 46 patients with sporting injuries to the knee. The ibuprofen-treated groups showed increased joint mobility and weight-bearing capability when compared to a placebo-treated group, again demonstrating the usefulness of anti-inflammatory drug therapy in sporting injuries. In this trial only one subject reported moderate gastric upset and this was a patient in the high dose group. The normal recommended dose range for ibuprofen for musculoskeletal disorders is 600–1200 mg daily in three to four divided doses, preferably after food.

A maximum recommended dose for the drug is now 2400 mg daily although higher levels have been used on some occasions.

Indomethacin

Indomethacin has been used for treating inflammatory conditions since the mid-1960s and remains a very frequently prescribed drug. Whilst being an effective anti-inflammatory drug it does suffer, apart from the gastric irritant activity somewhat typical of this type of drug, from a number of central nervous system side effects such as headaches, dizziness and light headedness. Generally, indomethacin is found to be of similar efficacy to other non-steroidal anti-inflammatory drugs, such as naproxen, in the treatment of soft-tissue sports injuries. As might be expected, the drop-out rate due to the side effects of this drug is generally higher than for other members of this group using normal therapeutic doses of indomethacin (50–200 mg daily). As many as half the patients experience some untoward symptoms and many of these will have to withdraw from using the drug. The drug is normally initiated as 25 mg, two or three times daily and gradually increased if necessary. It is possible that at this low starting dose toxicity is less of a problem. Edwards *et al.* (1984) found it necessary to withdraw only one patient from a group of 53 who were receiving 75 mg indomethacin daily for acute soft tissue sports injuries. Indomethacin is also available in 50 mg suppositories for night time use and these may be of benefit in some individuals.

Piroxicam

Piroxicam is one of the newest anti-inflammatory agents to become generally available. It is often difficult to assess the place of a particular drug in the field of therapy until considerable experience has been obtained with it. Initial results suggest that it is comparable to indomethacin or naproxen in treating acute musculoskeletal injuries but that it is better tolerated than aspirin or indomethacin. One particular advantage of piroxicam is that it has a long half-life which permits its use as a single daily dose, usually of 20 mg. There has been concern recently that piroxicam is more ulcerogenic than other aspirin-like drugs and these concerns have been widely reported in the popular press. The Committee on Safety of Medicines and the Drug Surveillance Research Unit in Britain have concluded that large and clinically important differences in rates of gastrointestinal bleeding, perforation and ulceration between piroxicam and other aspirin-like drugs probably do not exist.

Phenylbutazone

Phenylbutazone was introduced into clinical medicine in 1949 to take its place alongside the salicylates for the treatment of arthritic conditions. It is a powerful anti-inflammatory drug and is capable of treating acute exacerbations of rheumatoid arthritis and severe ankylosing spondylitis (an inflammatory condition of the spine). Compared to the many newer anti-inflammatory agents now available it is subject to a large number of toxic side effects some of which have led to fatal outcomes. Whilst many physicians believe this to be an extraordinarily useful anti-inflammatory agent others have argued that it is too dangerous to use. The most serious side effects are undoubtedly the retention of fluid, which in predisposed individuals may precipitate cardiac failure, and the interference with normal blood cell production most commonly resulting in aplastic anaemia and agranulocytosis which can occur within the first few days of treatment. Its use, therefore, in trivial, self-limiting musculoskeletal disorders is difficult to justify. In the UK, phenylbutazone is now only indicated for the treatment of ankylosing spondylitis in hospital situations and its closely related congener oxyphenbutazone has been withdrawn completely. By contrast, in the US it is still widely used, and a report by Marshall (1979) states that in the National Football League, for example, an average of 24–40 unit doses of phenylbutazone are used per player per season. The treatment of sports injuries is not, however, a licensed indication for Butazolidin (phenylbutazone) in the USA.

Whatever the role of phenylbutazone in injuries in sportsmen and sportswomen, there is no doubt that it is used considerably in the field of equestrian sports. In show jumping the horses' feet are subjected to constant concussion. By the age of 10, many show jumping horses will have suffered pathological changes in their feet but in many cases will be at their peak. Similarly, three day event horses are subject to considerable physical stress with strain of a tendon or the suspensory ligament being common injuries. Even without jumping-related competition, the regular galloping activity, as in, for example, flat racing or polo, may result in substantial changes in bones, joints and ligaments of a horse and when pushed too hard or for too long lameness may develop due to the pain and inflammation of the particular injury. The time-honoured remedy for reducing the pain and inflammation of these injuries in horses is to administer an anti-inflammatory drug the most frequently used being phenylbutazone.

Horses generally tolerate phenylbutazone very well and may be treated with the drug to improve their comfort. Whilst there are many indications for the use of phenylbutazone in horses, dilemmas do arise as to whether their use may mask an injury and lead to a complete breakdown of an affected limb. The governing bodies of equestrian sports generally recognize the usefulness of this drug but exclude the use of the drug on, or immediately before, competition days in order that no unfair advantage may be gained by improving performance and also to protect unfit horses from being used competitively.

3.4.3 PROTEOLYTIC ENZYMES AS ANTI-INFLAMMATORY AGENTS

Several reports have been published suggesting that proteolytic enzyme preparations are useful for the treatment of soft-tissue sports injuries. Hyaluronidase, which splits the glucosaminidic bonds of hyaluronic acid, reduces the viscosity of the cellular cement. Local injections of this enzyme have been shown to reduce the healing time of sprained ankles. Chymotrypsin preparations which are available in tablet form have also been found to be useful in sporting injuries. Whilst these enzymes are obviously vulnerable to gastrointestinal breakdown, there is evidence that some active enzyme is absorbed. A number of clinical trials have been conducted amongst professional players of association football and whilst not all have shown favourable results, some trials have found a significant reduction in recovering time to match fitness, particularly where haematomata or sprains were the major feature of the injury. In one notable trial, where an enzyme preparation was compared with placebo in a London club, the physicians monitoring the trial were so impressed by the apparent efficacy of the enzyme that the trial was abandoned since it was considered unjustifiable to withhold the enzyme from the placebo group. This was deemed especially so since the club was in the running for major honours that season!

Here we have an enigma. On the one hand, we have apparently convincing reports that proteolytic enzyme preparations aid recovery from sports injury. On the other hand, we are faced with the fact that the bulk of these reports are over 20 years old. If these preparations could significantly reduce recovery time and return players to match fitness in perhaps only 70% of the normal time it should take, why are they not used? Perhaps the initial optimistic reports have not been subsequently reproducible or perhaps toxicity has limited their use; it is true that occasionally serious hypersensitivity reactions do occur. Whilst not now used for treating mechanically-induced trauma these preparations are regularly used in a variety of post-surgical situations to reduce oedema.

3.4.4 ANTI-INFLAMMATORY STEROIDS

Without question the most powerful anti-inflammatory agents known to man are the glucocorticoids. These are drugs which are based on the chemical structure of adrenal corticosteroids. In 1949, Hench and his colleagues demonstrated the beneficial effects of high doses of cortisone in patients with rheumatoid arthritis. Considerable interest was generated in this hormone as a potential cure for inflammatory disorders but it rapidly became apparent that this substance was not curative and that it had no lasting effect on the disease process. More potent activity was found in hydrocortisone (cortisol) the predominant glucocorticoid secreted in man. The anti-inflammatory activity of these steroid hormones appears to be secondary to their glucocorticoid function as despite the severe metabolic derangement which accompanies adrenal gland insufficiency (Addison's disease) there is no general precipitation of inflammatory reactions. Many attempts have been made to increase the anti-inflammatory activity of these steroids. A large number of anti-inflammatory steroids are now available, many of which are an order of magnitude more potent than cortisol but all have significant glucocorticoid activity. This limits their long-term use because they disturb the metabolic activity of the body in much the same way as occurs in conditions of hyperactive secretion of the adrenal cortex (Cushing's syndrome). It is, therefore, important that a distinction is made between the long-term use of anti-inflammatory steroids and their use in acute situations. The long-term use of these drugs may lead to a number of side effects, some of which may be particularly unfortunate for an athlete. Osteoporosis is frequently encountered during corticosteroid therapy. This serious weakening of the skeletal structure principally affects those bones with the most trabecular structure such as the ribs and vertebrae and vertebral compression fractures are a frequent complication of steroid therapy. Long-term use of a drug, which may weaken the bone structure of an individual whose activities may subject that structure to greater than normal stress should not be contemplated lightly. Perhaps a more significant problem, however, is the catabolic effect of glucocorticoids on skeletal muscle. Weakness of muscles in the arms and legs can occur soon after treatment is started, even with quite modest doses of these anti-inflammatory drugs. Experiments with ráts have shown that very signficant reductions in muscle weight can occur within seven days of treatment. Interestingly the effect is restricted to skeletal muscle with cardiac muscle being noticeably spared. If long-term systemic steroid treatment is initiated it must be realized that as well as the anti-inflammatory effect which will be achieved, the administered drug will largely take over the glucocorticoid role of the natural adrenal hormone. Due to negative feedback mechanisms operating in both the hypothalamus and the anterior pituitary, the release of adrenocorticotrophic hormone is inhibited and so the adrenal cortex is not stimulated to produce its own glucocorticoids normally. Over a period of time the adrenal cortex regresses to a state such that if the drug treatment is stopped suddenly the adrenal gland can no longer respond to the demands placed on it and fails to produce sufficient quantities of glucocorticoid. It is important, therefore, that following long-term treatment with a steroid, the drug is only gradually withdrawn by a progressive lowering of the daily dose.

Steroids are double-edged weapons in the armoury of anti-inflammatory therapy. They are very powerful anti-inflammatory drugs but they are, unfortunately, likely to cause a great many side effects. The direct application of these drugs to an affected site so that a high concentration of the steroid is achieved locally but not systemically offers the possibility of gaining the maximum usefulness of steroids with minimal toxicity. Direct application of steroids to the skin is not an entirely satisfactory method as although they are generally well absorbed large proportions of the active drug will be transported away by the blood and, therefore, accumulation in affected muscle or connective tissue is limited. Additionally, topical application of steroids tends to cause thinning of the skin and a slowing down of wound healing. The local injection of a corticosteroid preparation does offer considerable advantages in the treatment of an inflammatory condition restricted to a small area of the body. Early attempts to inject steroids locally were not particularly successful as these highly soluble drugs were rapidly redistributed from the site. The development of less soluble esters of hydrocortisone and prednisolone to give fairly insoluble microcyrstal-line preparations which are injected as suspensions has markedly

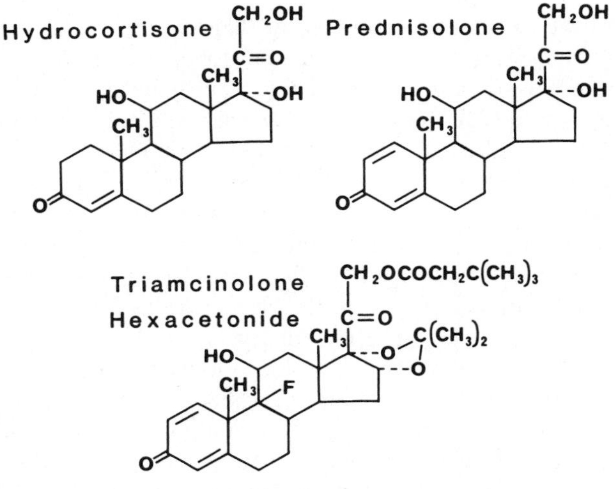

Figure 3.4 Some examples of anti-inflammatory steroids.

improved the success of this particular technique. A single dose of an insoluble steroid preparation will provide relief for several days or even several weeks. If necessary, these local injections can be repeated to extend the period of effectiveness. Great care must be taken when injections of steroids are given to minimize the risk of the introducton of infective agents. This is especially the case where injections have to be administered intra-articularly to improve mobility and restrict damage of an affected joint. In the case of intra-articular injection, the use of a long-acting preparation such as triamcinalone hexacetonide is indicated so that repeated injections are less necessary, or at least, less frequent (Figure 3.4).

Local injections of steroids are also valuable for the treatment of soft tissue injuries. They may be injected into the interior of a bursa (the fibrous sac filled with synovial fluid which may be found between muscles or between a tendon and bone, and which facilitates frictionless movement between the surfaces that it separates); they may also be injected into a tendon sheath to reduce the inflammation of an affected tendon or infiltrated around the area of an inflamed ligament. Tendinitis of the elbow (tennis elbow) is a classical example of the type of injury which responds well to local corticosteroid injection.

Steroids do have the property of delaying the wound healing process and so particular care should be taken in their use when extensive new tissue will have to be produced to repair damage, for example, where collision on the sports field has led to an open wound. In this instance the use of steroids to reduce inflammation may not be appropriate. The means by which these steroids extend their anti-inflammatory effects is not clear. It is probable that they have a number of activities, all of which contribute to their anti-inflammatory effects. They have been shown to reduce the output of chemical mediators of inflammation and to inhibit the effects of mediators on the vascular endothelium resulting in a reduction of oedema formation. They have also been shown to have a number of inhibitory actions on the responsiveness of white blood cells. They are, for example, particularly effective in reducing the activity of thymocytes which are involved with delayed hypersensitivity reactions. Whatever their mechanism of action, and despite the potential hazards of long-term, high dose therapy, glucocorticoids are profoundly effective in the reduction of inflammatory reactions and their place in the treatment of sporting injuries is assured.

3.5 References and further reading

Andersen, L. A. and Gotzsche, P. C. (1984) Naproxen and aspirin in acute musculoskeletal disorders: a double-blind, parallel study in patients with sports injuries. *Pharmactherpeutica*, 3, 531.

Bonta, I. L., Bult, H., Vincent, J. E. and Ziglstra, F. J. (1977) Acute anti-inflammatory effects of aspirin and dexamethasone in rats deprived of endogenous prostaglandin precursors. *J. Pharm. Pharmacol.*, 29, 1.

Boyne, P. S. and Medhurst, H. (1967) Oral anti-inflammatory enzyme therapy in injuries in professional footballers. *Practitioner*, 198, 543.

Bullock, G. J., Carter, E. E., Elliott, P., Peters, R. F., Simpson, P. and White, A. M. (1971) Relative changes in the function of muscle ribosomes, and mitochondria during the early phase of steroid-induced catabolism. *Biochem. J.*, 127, 881.

Crook, D., Collins, A. J., Bacon, P. A. and Chan, R. (1976) Prostaglandin synthetase activity from human rheumatoid synovial microsomes. *Ann. Rheum. Dis.*, 35, 327.

Edwards, V., Wilson, A. A., Harwood, H. F. *et al.* (1984) A multicentre comparison of piroxicam and indomethacin in acute soft tissue sports injuries. *J. Int. Med. Res.*, 12, 46.

Ferreira, S. H., Moncada, S. and Vane, J. R. (1971) Indomethacin and aspirin abolish prostaglandin release from the spleen. *Nature*, 231, 232.

Flower, R. J., Moncada, S. and Vane, J. R. (1985) Analgesic-antipyretics and anti-inflammatory agents; drugs employed in the treatment of gout. In

Goodman and Gilman's The Pharmacological Basis of Therapeutics 7th edn (eds A. G. Gilman, L. S. Goodman, T. W. Rall, F. Murad), Macmillan, London.

Haynes, R. C. Jr and Murad, F. (1985) Adrenocortictropic hormone; adrenocortical steroids and their synthetic analogs; inhibitors of adrenocortical steroid biosynthesis. In *Goodman and Gilman's The Pharmacological Basis of Therapeutics* 7th edn (eds A. G. Gilman, L. S. Goodman, T. W. Rall, F. Murad), Macmillan, London.

Hench, P. S., Kendall, E. C., Slocumb, C. H. and Polley, H. F. (1949) The effect of a hormone on the adrenal cortex (17-hydroxy-11-dehydrocorticosterone: compound E) and of pituitary adrenocorticotropic hormone on rheumatoid arthritis. *Proc. Staff Meet. Mayo Clinic*, **24**, 181.

Hutson, M. A. (1986) A double-blind study comparing ibuprofen 1800 mg or 2400 mg daily and placebo in sports injuries. *J. Int. Med. Res.*, **4**, 142.

Lewis, T. (1927) *The Blood Vessels of the Human Skin and their Responses*. Shaw and Sons, London.

MacLagan, T. (1876) The treatment of acute rheumatism by salacin. *Lancet*, i, 342.

Marshall, E. (1979) Drugging of football players curbed by central monitoring plan, NFL claims. *Science*, **203**, 626.

Moncada, S., Flower, R. J. and Vane, J. R. (1985) Prostaglandin, prostacyclin, thromboxane A_2 and leukotrienes. In *Goodman and Gilman's Pharmacological Basis of Therapeutics*, 7th edn (eds A. G. Gilman, L. S. Goodman, T. W. Rall, F. Murad), Macmillan, London.

Ryan, G. B. and Majno, G. (1977) *Inflammation*. Upjohn Company, Kalamazoo, Michigan.

Smith, J. B. and Willis, A. L. (1971) Aspirin selectively inhibits prostaglandin production in human platelets. *Nature*, **231**, 235.

Vane, J. R. (1971) Inhibition of prostaglandin synthesis as a mechanism of action for aspirin-like drugs. *Nature*, **231**, 232.

4   Central nervous system stimulants

A. J. GEORGE

Various drugs which stimulate the central nervous system (CNS) have been known for over 2000 years. A simple classification of these substances is complicated by their combination of central and systemic effects. Thus, though the compounds mainly stimulate CNS activity many central stimulants have, in addition, direct effects on cardiovascular functions and on the sympathetic nervous system.

4.1 CNS neurophysiology

To understand the various mechanisms by which CNS stimulants produce their effects, it is necessary to understand the basic functioning of neurones in the CNS (Figure 4.1). The stimulant drug must pass from the circulation, across the blood–brain barrier and into the brain tissue spaces. Once in the brain it may: (a) increase neurotransmitter release onto receptors (amphetamine and ephedrine); (b) directly stimulate the post-synaptic receptors (ephedrine, caffeine); (c) inhibit neurotransmitter re-uptake (cocaine and amphetamine).

CNS stimulants are thought to act mainly on the dopamine (DA), noradrenaline (NA) and 5 hydroxytryptamine (5HT) neurotransmitter systems. Caffeine is thought to affect adenosine neurotransmission.

4.2 Amphetamine

Several structurally related drugs are known as 'amphetamines' and include dextroamphetamine, methamphetamine, phenmetrazine and

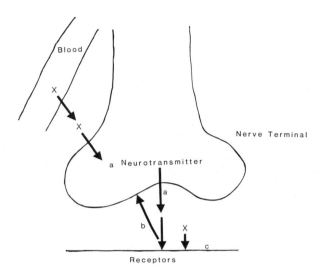

Figure 4.1 Sites of action of CNS stimulants. (a) amphetamine; (b) amphetamine and cocaine; (c) caffeine.

methylphenidate. In this chapter the word amphetamine will refer to dextroamphetamine, the structure of which is shown in Figure 4.2.

Amphetamine is a phenyl isopropylamine (Figure 4.2) and was first synthesized in 1920. It was originally prescribed for the treatment of nasal congestion – inhalation of an amphetamine spray through the nose induced nasal vasoconstriction which resulted in decongestion. In 1935, amphetamine was first used to treat the neurological condition narcolepsy, and its use in the treatment of depression, anxiety and hyperactivity in children followed from this. Amphetamine was used widely during the Second World War to reduce fatigue and increase alertness particularly amongst naval and airforce crew on patrol duties. An indirect reference to this is made in Montserrat's *The Cruel Sea*. The rapid development of tolerance to amphetamine and the insidious occurrence of dependence have led to the drug being withdrawn from clinical use except in certain controlled circumstances.

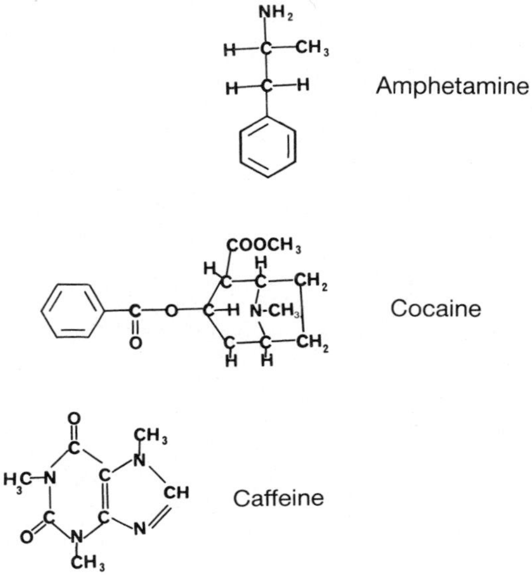

Figure 4.2 The structures of some CNS stimulants.

4.2.1 THE EFFECT OF AMPHETAMINES ON HUMAN MOOD AND PERFORMANCE

The desire to enhance mood or performance or both is usually the main reason for taking amphetamines. In their comprehensive review of amphetamines Weiss and Laties (1962) agreed that amphetamine does produce an enhanced performance in many tasks and does not simply normalize fatigue responses. They examined various tasks such as (a) work output by subjects on a bicycle ergometer, (b) performance on arduous military exercises, and (c) performance during flying or driving missions. Apparent improvements in athletic performance in events as diverse as shot put, swimming and running are produced by amphetamines as well as a reduction in reaction time and increased coordination and steadiness. These aspects will be discussed in detail later. Intellectual performance does not seem to be improved by amphetamines, unless the performance has been degraded by boredom and fatigue (Brookes, 1985). In the short term, amphetamine increases the speed of learning of new tasks. The effects of amphetamine on judgement are uncertain and several conflicting studies have been published (Brookes, 1985). There is general agreement that amphetamines cause a mild distortion of time perception which may lead to misjudgement in planning maneouvres or in manipulations such as driving a car. Active avoidance learning is facilitated by amphetamine. Although there is considerable inter-individual variation in the effects of amphetamine on mood the general effects are of positive mood enhancement. These positive effects include an increase in physical energy, mental aptitude, talkativeness, restlessness, excitement and good humour. Subjects taking amphetamine also report that they feel confident, efficient, ambitious and that their food intake is reduced.

Some 'negative' effects of amphetamine include anxiety, indifference, slowness in reasoning, irresponsible behaviour, irritability and restlessness, dry mouth, tremors, insomnia and following withdrawal, depression. These effects of amphetamine on mood are dose-dependent and are thought to be produced by the stimulation of dopamine and noradrenergic receptors.

Tolerance and dependence

Tolerance develops rapidly to many of the effects of the amphetamines. Tolerance is said to be present when, over a period of time, increasing doses of a drug are required to maintain the same response. Brookes (1985) has reported several cases of subjects requiring as much as 1 g of amphetamine per day to produce the same effect on mood as a new taker of amphetamines who may require only 10–30 mg. There is much evidence to show that amphetamines induce drug dependence and the amphetamine-dependent person may become psychotic (see p. 114), aggressive and anti-social. Withdrawal of amphetamines is associated with mental and physical depression.

4.2.2 THERAPEUTIC USE

The many varied uses of amphetamine following its original introduction are now largely discredited. It is interesting to compare the initial enthusiasm for amphetamine as the 'cure-all' for numerous mental problems with that for the use of cocaine some 50 years previously.

Until quite recently amphetamine was used to treat narcolepsy but its use is now limited to the treatment of hyperactivity in childen. A rare use of amphetamines is as a disgnostic aid in determining which patients are unsuitable for a particular anti-manic or anti-schizophrenic treatment.

Toxicity

The major side effects of amphetamine administration (excluding those following withdrawal of the drug) include (a) many of the negative effects described previously; (b) confusion, delirium, sweating, palpitations, dilation of the pupil and rapid breathing; (c) hypertension, tachycardia, tremors, muscle and joint pain. Though amphetamines may initially stimulate libido, chronic amphetamine use often leads to a reduction in sex drive. Chronic amphetamine administration is also associated with myocardial pathology and also with growth retardation in adolescents. Usually the personality changes induced by chronic low doses of amphetamine are gradually reversed after the drug is stopped. However, high chronic doses may lead to a variety of persistent personality changes. Possibly the most serious of the severe personality disorders induced by amphetamine is the so-called amphetamine psychosis described by Connell in 1958. The frightening array of psychiatric symptoms he described in patients presenting with amphetamine psychosis include many commonly found in paranoid type schizophrenics. An important distinction between amphetamine psychosis and schizophrenia is that amphetamine induces a preponderance of symptoms of paranoid and of visual hallucinations.

4.2.3 THE MODE OF ACTION OF AMPHETAMINE

There are four main mechanisms by which amphetamine may produce its effects. These are (1) release of neurotransmitter – dopamine, noradrenaline or 5HT – from their respective nerve terminals; (2) inhibition of monoamine oxidase activity; (3) inhibition of neurotransmitter re-uptake; and (4) direct action on neurotransmitter receptors. Of these four possibilities, neurotransmitter release appears to be the most important (Brookes, 1985). It seems that several major behavioural changes induced by amphetamine are most closely mimicked by stimulation of central noradrenaline-releasing neurones. Thus, the amphetamine induced locomotor activity and self-stimulation seen in animals and the increased alertness and elevation of mood produced in humans are closely related to increases in noradrenergic activity. Amphetamine is a potent anorectic and elevates plasma free fatty acid levels. Body temperature is also elevated. The cardiovascular, gastrointestinal and respiratory effects of amphetamine are sympatho-mimetic in nature. However, both animal and clinical experiments suggest that the effects of amphetamine are mediated by the release of at least two neurotransmitters NA and DA and that in the rat the development of tolerance to amphetamine involves the release of 5HT. In particular, the stereotyped behaviour induced in the rat by amphet-amine administration appears to depend on DA release. The euphoriant action of amphetamine can be abolished by the DA receptor antagonist pimozide. There is some evidence to suggest that the positive behavioural effects of amphetamine may be mediated by DA while the effect of amphetamine on food intake may be mediated by NA. However, Silverstone and Goodall (1985) produced conflicting evi-dence of this.

Pharmacokinetics

Amphetamines are readily absorbed, mainly from the small intestine and the peak plasma concentration occurs in 1–2 hours following administration. Absorption is usually complete in 2.5–4 hours and is accelerated by food intake.

The metabolism of amphetamines has been difficult to investigate because of the wide variation between species in the metabolic effects of amphetamines. The principle amphetamine metabolites are p-hydroxy ephedrine and p-hydroxyamphetamine. Both these metabolites have similar pharmacological effects to the parent amphetamine. Amphet-amine is lost from the blood by renal filtration. Some secretion of amphetamine into the urine also occurs. Amphetamine excretion is enhanced by an acid urine and treatments which increase the acidity of urine enhance amphetamine loss – a reaction which is useful in the treatment of amphetamine overdose.

4.2.4 THE EFFECTS OF AMPHETAMINE IN SPORT

In the USA, the increasing use of amphetamines in all sports led the American Medical Association to initiate research projects to test the effects of amphetamine on sports performance and the incidence of side effects associated with the drug. One of these studies (Smith and Beecher, 1959) reported that 14–21 mg of amphetamine sulphate per kg body weight when administered 2–3 hours prior to running, swimming or weight throwing, improved performance in 75% of the cases investigated. This was a double-blind study in which 14 out of 15 swimmers and 19 out of 26 runners showed a statistically significant improvement in performance after amphetamine administration. However, the improvements demonstrated were quite small (usually 1%). This study also demonstrated that the performance of athletes in throwing events was improved by an average of 4% following amphetamine administration. Criticism of the study soon followed because the athletes were sometimes allowed to time themselves, there was little control for weather conditions and, a wide range of distances (600 yards to 12 miles) was used to test the athletes and a minor dosage of amphetamine was administered. Chandler and Blair (1980) reported that amphetamine improved athletic performance in terms of acceleration, knee extension strength and time to exhaustion but that it had no effect on sprinting speed.

Haldi and Wynn (1959) reported that 5 mg of amphetamine 90 minutes before a 100 yard swim had no effect on the time of the swim. A more sophisticated double-blind investigation of amphetamine was carried out by Golding and Barnard (1963) using a treadmill. They studied the effect of amphetamine on treadmill running in trained and untrained subjects. Each subject undertook an initial run followed 12 minutes later by a second 'fatigued' run. Thus, the effects of amphetamine on initial performance and fatigue could be examined in the same subject. Their results showed that amphetamine had no effect on performance during the initial and fatigued runs in either the trained or the untrained athletes. During the fatigued runs, amphetamine retarded the recovery rates for heart rate and blood pressure. Only one of the subjects was able to tell that he was receiving amphetamine. Many of the studies on the effects of amphetamine on athletic performance have been carried out on cyclists. One reason for this is that there are numerous examples of fatalities arising from the use of amphetamines by cyclists, notably the incidence of death from heatstroke. Wyndham et al. (1971) carried out a wide-ranging placebo controlled biochemical and physiological investigation on two champion cyclists exercising on a bicycle ergometer. While working at rates between 12 000 and 16 000 ft lb.min^{-1} there was no difference between amphetamine and placebo in terms of submaximal or maximal oxygen uptake, heart rate or minute ventilation; however, there were signficant increases in blood lactate levels. The authors concluded that amphetamines have no effect on the ability to do aerobic work but they insignificantly increased the cyclists ability to tolerate higher levels of anaerobic metabolism. The dangers inherent in these results are that an athlete taking amphetamine might be better able to ignore the usual internal signals of over-exertion and heat stress which may therefore explain the incidence of heatstroke and cardiac problems in cyclists who take amphetamines during long-distance cycling events.

Since no significant improvement in performance is associated with amphetamine use, why does it continue to be taken? The answer could be an effect on mental attitude in terms of improved mood, greater confidence and optimism and increased alertness. It is also possible that amphetamine might increase preparedness and make the athlete more keyed up for his event. To examine this possibility the effects of amphetamine sulphate were compared with the tranquillizer meprobamate and with placebo control in 26 male medical students. The results showed that none of the students was able to tell which drug he was taking and also there was no correlation between either subjective feelings of increased alertness in those taking amphetamine or lethargy in subjects on meprobamate, with any change in reaction time or manipulative skills (Golding, 1981).

Several studies thus indicate that the effect of amphetamine on the psychological state of athletes is almost certainly self-induced and occurs as a result of the athlete expecting to perform better and to be more alert.

Side effects of amphetamine in relation to sport

Some particular side effects of amphetamine are particularly important in athletes and have often only been revealed in individuals undertaking extremely arduous training or sporting schedules.

One of the most widely publicised side effects of amphetamine from which a number of fatalities have occurred is heat stroke. This has been most prominent in cyclists owing to the intensity of their exercise, the endurance required, and the high ambient temperatures at which the exercise often occurs. Amphetamine causes a redistribution of blood flow away from the skin, thus limiting the cooling of the blood. As a result of this, two cyclists (Jenson and Simpson) who had both been taking amphetamine died of heatstroke and cardiac arrest respectively during gruelling road races. The former occurred in the intense summer heat of Rome, the latter whilst climbing the infamous Mont Ventoux during the 1967 Tour de France.

The ability of amphetamines to obscure painful injuries has enabled many American footballers to play on and exacerbate injuries which would normally have resulted in their withdrawal from play.

The side effects of amphetamine on behaviour are also important in sport. Mandell (1979) has investigated amphetamine abuse amongst American footballers and found extensive abuse amounting to 60–70 mg average dose per man per game. In this sport, amphetamine was administered apparently to promote aggression and weaken fatigue in the footballers. However, there are several accounts quoted by Golding (1981) in which the euphoriant effects of such doses have rendered the takers unaware of the errors and misjudgements they were making on the pitch.

Why take amphetamines?

Why take amphetamines when the chance of increased injury, dependence, heatstroke and cardiac arrest is enhanced by these drugs and the actual improvement on performance, if it does occur, is so small – in the order of 1 or 2%? The simple answer to this was proposed by Laties and Weiss (1981) who examined the improvements in world records in athletic events over the past 100 years. As an example, the 1500 m world record has improved by only 15% since 1880 and on average in the past 50 years it has improved by only 1% in every 7 years. Thus, they concluded that a top athlete who could consistently maintain a 1% improvement in performance would be at an advantage over competitors. This advantage they termed 'the amphetamine margin'.

4.2.5 CONCLUSION

The prescription and administration of amphetamines are strictly controlled by law in most developed countries. They produce powerful stimulating effects on the CNS, which include euphoria, excitation and increased aggression and alertness. These effects are achieved at the expense of judgement and self-criticism. Amphetamine administration may be followed by severe bouts of depression and dependence. Increases in athletic performance induced by amphetamine are very small and several studies have failed to show that amphetamine produces any physical advantage. Some evidence suggests that amphetamine may increase confidence before and during an event and laboratory studies have shown that it may also reduce fatigue in isometric muscle contraction.

The induction of dependence and the increased susceptibility to heatstroke and cardiac abnormalities seem to suggest that amphetamine taking is of little value as a performance-enhancing drug.

4.3 Cocaine

This alkaloid occurs naturally in the leaf of the coca plant (Erythroxylon coca) which grows in a wide area of Central and South America. South American Indians, particularly the Incas, chewed the leaf as an aid to digestion and to help them with arduous work at high altitudes. In the last century, pure cocaine was extracted and isolated. The pure drug was popularized by, among others, Sigmund Freud as a suggested 'cure-all' for many mental disorders. After several tragic accidents and following the addiction of many patients to the drug, cocaine was used subsequently only as a local anaesthetic. The drug is now prescribed only as a euphoriant when it is administered concurrently with morphine as a pain palliative in terminal illness.

4.3.1 PHARMACOLOGY

Cocaine is a powerful inhibitor of the re-uptake of NA and DA into their respective nerve terminals. Recently, cocaine has been shown to antagonize 5HT receptors. Thus stimulation by cocaine increases the potency of noradrenaline and dopamine at their respective post-synaptic sites. There is some evidence that cocaine may increase the release of NA and DA from their respective nerve terminals. After administration it is rapidly converted in the liver and plasma to several water soluble metabolites, such as ecgonine.

4.3.2 CNS EFFECTS

These are thought to be due to the effects on dopamine and not noradrenaline but the exact mechanism by which cocaine induces its effects is unknown. In animal behaviour experiments involving self-administration cocaine is one of the most powerful reinforcing agents. In humans, cocaine causes euphoria, increased alertness and a feeling of increased power both mental and physical. When interviewed, cocaine abusers say that cocaine has become the most important feature of their lives. As a corollary, animals allowed to self-administer cocaine no longer drink, eat, sleep or copulate.

Adverse effects

These are mainly seen in the CNS and respiratory system. General adverse effects include agitation, restlessness, insomnia and anxiety. A 'cocaine psychosis' is associated with chronic cocaine abuse and is characterized by hallucinations which may be auditory, visual, olfactory, tactile or paranoid.

Sniffing cocaine leads to chronic rhinitis and in heavy abusers septal necrosis may occur. Since cocaine potentiates the action of NA and DA many of the peripheral systems regulated by the sympathetic nervous system are likely to be involved. Thus, cocaine potentiates NA effects on the heart and on the vascular system.

4.3.3 EFFECTS IN ATHLETES

Because of the dangers inherent in cocaine administration and the strength and rapidity of onset of dependence no studies of the effects of cocaine on athletic performance have been carried out. However, the major groups in the USA who have been associated with cocaine abuse are footballers and cyclists.

Adverse effects in athletes

The central affects have already been discussed generally.

The specific peripheral effects of importance to athletes are increased cardiac activity and cardiac sensitivity to stimulation and reduced thermoregulatory efficiency. In terms of the cardiovascular system, cocaine potentiates the action of NA and adrenaline on the heart producing arrhythmias, tachycardia and hypertension. Possibly the most dramatic and life-threatening effect of cocaine is coronary occlusion which was almost certainly the cause of death in two cases, involving a basketball player and a footballer, which are discussed in detail by Cantwell and Rose (1981). They also describe the recovery of a 21-year-old cocaine-abusing athlete from a coronary occlusion following combined amphetamine and cocaine abuse.

Table 4.1 Caffeine content of some beverages, drinks and medicines

	Caffeine content (mg)
Coffee (per 5 oz cup)	
Percolated	64–124
Instant	40–108
Filter	110–150
Decaffeinated	2–5
Tea (per 5 oz cup)	
1 minute brew	9–33
5 minute brew	25–50
Soft drinks (per 12 oz serving)	
Pepsi Cola	38.4
Coca Cola	46
Proprietary medicines	
Anadin tablet	15
Cephos tablet	10
Coldrex cold treatment tablet	25
Phensic tablet	50

4.3.4 CONCLUSION

A thorough scientific evaluation of the effects of cocaine on athletic performance is impossible because of medical, ethical and legal considerations. It appears that whatever sporting advantage might be gained by cocaine use is far outweighed by the serious cardiovascular side effects which the drug produces.

4.4 Caffeine

The three psychoactive drugs most commonly used are alcohol, nicotine and caffeine and all are self-administered! It has been suggested that caffeine has been in use as a stimulant since the stone age! Caffeine is a member of the methyl xanthine group of compounds which also includes theophylline and theobromine. Caffeine occurs naturally in coca, coffee beans and tea leaves. The amount of caffeine obtained from each source depends on the method of extraction and the particle size of the extracts. Caffeine is added to soft drinks such as the many types of colas and is also present in a number of 'over the counter' medicines (Table 4.1).

4.4.1 PHARMACOLOGY

Caffeine usually exerts an effect on the CNS in doses ranging from 85 to 200 mg and in this dose range it produces a reduction in drowsiness and fatigue, an elevation in mood, improved alertness and productivity, increased capacity for sustained intellectual effort and a rapid and clearer flow of thought. This dose range of caffeine also causes diuresis, a relaxation of smooth muscle, activation of gastric acid secretion and an increase in heart rate, blood pressure and blood vessel diameter. A caffeine dose in excess of 250 mg is considered to be high and may cause headaches, instability and nervousness. The American Psychiatric Association considers caffeine intoxication as occurring at doses greater than 250 mg. Caffeine is readily absorbed from the gastrointestinal tract and is rapidly distributed throughout all tissues and organs. Peak blood levels are reached within 15–45 minutes after oral administration in man, although the type of drink may affect the absorption rate. For example, caffeine is absorbed more slowly from Coca Cola than from tea or coffee. The plasma half-life, that is the time for a given concentration in the plasma to reduce by half, varies among individuals (range 3–10 hours). In smokers, caffeine is removed from the plasma much more rapidly than in the non-smoker, while in women taking oral contraceptives the half-life of caffeine is doubled.

Many athletes are convinced that caffeine improves their performance, while many a student (and this author) have improved their mental concentration by taking drinks containing caffeine. These uses aside, it must be remembered that caffeine consumption (as coffee) has been associated with a number of systemic disorders which include hypertension, myocardial infarction, peptic ulcer and cancers of the gastrointestinal tract and urinary tract.

4.4.2 THE EFFECTS OF CAFFEINE

Caffeine causes:

1. Increased gastric acid and pepsin secretion plus increased secretion into the small intestine.

2. Increased heart rate, stroke volume, cardiac output and blood pressure at rest.
3. Tachycardia.
4. Increased lipolysis.
5. Increased contractility of skeletal muscles.
6. Increased oxygen consumption and metabolic rate.
7. Increased diuresis.

Central effects

Caffeine in 200–400 mg doses produced fewer attention lapses during a study of night driving in a motor rally but it was shown that as the plasma caffeine level declines a rebound drowsiness may occur. Caffeine is said to counteract the reduction in performance caused by fatigue or boredom but there is no clear evidence that it can increase performance above control levels.

Some researchers have found positive evidence of the enhancement of mental performance by caffeine. Other workers have found no significant effect of caffeine on numerical reasoning, verbal fluency, short-term memory or digital skill. This conflict in findings may be due to differences in personality, i.e. extroverts may react differently to introverts. Dividing subjects up on the basis of their impulsiveness shows that the effects of caffeine may vary with the time of day. Also an individual's normal pattern of caffeine consumption may have a bearing on the result.

The exact nature of the effects of caffeine on psychomotor behaviour remains to be defined but many studies show that it has a significant effect on assessment and measurement of mental performance.

Caffeine can interfere with the quality and quantity of normal sleep and such sleep disturbances resemble those reported by insomniacs. Coffee disturbs sleep EEG patterns and heavy coffee drinkers usually report a better sleep following a caffeine-free evening.

Adverse reactions

When coffee drinking became fashionable in Great Britain during the seventeenth century the effects of caffeine on behaviour were immediately noticed and there were suggestions that it should be banned. A high intake of caffeine can induce symptoms very similar to an anxiety neurosis. Caffeinism is (at least in the USA) a recognized medical syndrome characterized by anxiety, mood changes, sleep disruption and psychophysiological changes and withdrawal symptoms. A full range of symptoms including agitation, depression, gastrointestinal tract complaints, palpitations and arrythmias has been described by Greden (1974). The Diagnostic and Statistical Manual of Mental Disorders (DSM III) of the American Psychiatric Association describes caffeine intoxication as a condition simulating an anxiety attack in which the person experiences nausea, insomnia, restlessness and jitteriness. An intake of caffeine greater than 600 mg/day seems to produce depression and negative effects: the euphoriant effect of caffeine being seen at doses below this value.

Mechanism of action

Caffeine is a powerful inhibitor of the cyclic nucleotide phosphodiesterase enzymes. These enzymes inactivate the so-called intracellular 'second messengers' which are the link between receptor stimulation and cellular response. When these enzymes are inhibited, the action of intracellular messengers, such as cylic AMP, is increased. This is unlikely to be the mechanism of action of caffeine in the CNS, since the level of caffeine in the brain never reaches levels capable of inhibiting phosphodiesterases. The cardiac, renal and other peripheral effects of caffeine are probably mediated by this mechanism. Several researchers have demonstrated that caffeine is an antagonist of central adenosine receptors and this may well be its central mechanism of action as the central stimulatory activity of caffeine is correlated with its ability to bind to adenosine receptors (Daly, Butts-Lamb and Padgett, 1983).

4.4.3 EFFECTS IN ATHLETES

In 1965, Bellet, Kershbaum and Aspe described the elevation of blood fatty acids that occurred with caffeine ingestion. They concluded that caffeine improved endurance by enhancing fat utilization thus sparing glycogen stores. Using nine competitive cyclists, Costill, Dalsky and Fink (1978) studied the effects of caffeine on their general metabolism. Each cyclist exercised to exhaustion on a cycle ergometer at 50% of their aerobic capacity after ingesting either decaffeinated or normal coffee (containing 330 mg caffeine). The caffeine takers managed to exercise for 19.5% longer than the control group and also they had significantly higher levels of plasma fatty acids and blood glycerol. In the caffeine group, the respiratory quotient (RQ) was reduced, possibly indicating a shift from carbohydrate to fat utilization. It was suggested that increased lipolysis postponed exhaustion by slowing the rate of glycogen utilization in liver and skeletal muscle. Ivy, Costill and Fink (1979) found that caffeine increased work production in athletes by 7.4% compared to control conditions and in the same study fat oxidation was elevated by 31% during the last 70 minutes of the trial. Essig, Costill and Van Handel (1980) measured the effect of caffeine on insulin secretion and glycogen utilization in seven untrained male cyclists. Compared to controls, the caffeine group had a 51% increase in lipid oxidation. Muscle biopsies showed a 39% reduction in glycogen utilization. They concluded that caffeine ingestion can increase oxidation of fatty acids and glycerol in muscle. In contrast, Perkins and Williams (1975) could find no effect with 4, 7 or 10 mg of caffeine per kg body weight in 14 male students exercising to exhaustion. They found no significant difference between control and caffeine-taking groups in exercise time to exhaustion, even though there was a caffeine-induced increase in fatty acid level.

In general, studies show that caffeine has a positive ergogenic effect on large muscles and on short-term intense exercise which requires both strength and power. The moderate increase in performance produced by cocaine appears more predictable than with other CNS stimulants. Chronic utilization of caffeine seems likely to increase the risk of cardiovascular abnormalities and the blood concentration of caffeine which may be present in an athlete is limited by the various athletic authorities.

4.5 References

American Psychiatric Association (1980) *Diagnostic and Statistical Manual of Mental Disorders (DSMIII)*.

Bellet, S., Kershbaum, A. and Aspe, J. (1965) The effect of caffeine on free fatty acids. *Arch. Intern. Med.*, **116**, 750–2.

Brookes, L. G. (1985) Central nervous system stimulants. In *Psychopharmacology: Recent Advances and Future Prospects* (ed. S. D. Iverson), Oxford University Press, Oxford, pp. 264–77.

Cantwell, J. D. and Rose, F. D. (1981) Cocaine and cardiovascular events. *Physician and Sports Medicine*, **14**, 77–82.

Chandler, J. V. and Blair, S. N. (1980) The effect of amphetamines on selected physiological components related to athletic success. *Med. Sci. Sports Exerc.*, 12, 65–9.

Connell, P. H. (1958) *Amphetamine Psychosis*. Chapman and Hall, London.

Costill, D. L., Dalsky, G. P. and Fink, W. J. (1978) Effects of caffeine ingestion on metabolism and exercise performance. *Med. Sci. Sports*, 10, 155–8.

Daly, J. W., Butts-Lamb, P. and Padgett, W. (1983) Sub-classes of adenosine receptors in the central nervous system interaction with caffeine and related methyl xanthines. *Cell. Mol. Neurobiol.*, 3, 69–80.

Essig, D., Costill, D. L. and Van Handel, P. J. (1980) Effects of caffeine ingestion on utilisation of muscle glycogen and lipid during leg ergometer cycling. *Int. J. Sports Med.*, 1, 86–90.

Golding, L. A. (1981) Drugs and hormones. In *Ergogenic Aids and Muscular Performance* (ed. W. P. Morgan), Academic Press, London, pp. 368–97.

Golding, L. A. and Barnard, J. P. (1963) The effect of d-amphetamine sulphate on physical performance. *J. Sports Med.*, 3, 221–4.

Greden, J. F. (1974) Anxiety or caffeinism: a diagnostic dilemma. *Am. J. Psychiat.*, 131, 1089–92.

Haldi, J. and Wynn, W. (1959) Action of drugs on efficiency of swimmers. *Res. Quarterly*, 31, 449–553.

Ivy, J. L., Costill, D. L. and Fink, W. J. (1979) Influence of caffeine and carbohydrate feedings on endurance performance. *Med. Sci. Sports*, 11, 6–11.

Laties, V. G. and Weiss, B. (1981) The amphetamine margin in sports. Fed Proc 40 2689–2692.

Mandell, A. J. (1979) The Sunday syndrome: a unique pattern of amphetamine abuse indigenous to American Professional Football. *Clin. Toxicol.*, 15, 225–32.

Perkins, R. and Williams, M. H. (1975) Effects of caffeine upon maximal muscular endurance of females. *Med. Sci. Sports*, 7, 221–4.

Pierson, W. R., Rasch, P. J. and Brubaker, M. L. (1961) *Med. Sport*, 1, 61–6.

Silverstone, T. and Goodall, E. (1985) How amphetamine works. In *Psychopharmacology: Recent Advances and Future Prospects*, (ed. S. D. Iversen), Oxford University Press, Oxford, pp. 315–25.

Smith, G. M. and Beecher, H. G. (1959) Amphetamine sulphate and athletic performance. *JAMA.*, 170, 542–51.

Weiss, B. and Laties, V. G. (1962) Enhancement of human performance by caffeine and the amphetamines. *Pharmac. Rev.*, 14, 1–36.

Wyndham, G. H., Rogers, G. G., Benade, A. J. S. and Strydan, N. B. (1971) Physiological effects of the amphetamines during exercise. *S. Afr. Med. J.*, 45, 247–52.

5 Alcohol, anti-anxiety drugs and exercise

T. REILLY

5.1 Introduction

Throughout civilization and up to the present day human ingenuity has found various ways of coping with the stresses that life brings. Sometimes these entail a form of escapism into a drug-induced illusory world to eschew temporary troubles. A resort to alcohol, for example, can bring a transient euphoric uplift from pressing matters of the day. These strategies are perhaps truer today than they were in Dionysian cultures, exceptions being certain countries where alcohol is taboo for religious reasons. Indeed, it is generally believed that stress-induced illness is a phenomenon of contemporary urban civilization. The widespread prescription of tranquillisers and the high incidence of alcohol addiction support this view. Their impact on fitness and well-being has received scant attention.

Among athletes, participation in sports brings its own unique form of stress, usually before the more important contests. Though a certain amount of pre-competition anxiety is inevitable, the anxiety reaction varies enormously between individuals, with some coping extremely poorly. Many find their own solutions to attenuate anxiety levels, albeit sometimes with exogenous aids. Anxiety may adversely affect performance, especially in activities highly demanding of mental concentration and steadiness of limbs. This has prompted the use of anti-anxiety drugs, although some are not permitted in many sports.

In this chapter the relation between anxiety and sport performance is first explored. The next section concentrates on alcohol, its metabolism in the body and its effect on the central nervous system. The interactions

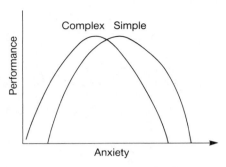

Figure 5.1 The relationship between level of anxiety and performance efficiency for simple and complex tasks.

between alcohol and health are then considered. Its impact on physiological responses to exercise and the uses in sport are then examined. The main 'minor' tranquillisers, the benzodiazepines, are discussed before finally the uses and abuses of other anti-anxiety drugs are described.

5.2 Anxiety and performance

The psychological reaction to impending sports competition is variously referred to as anxiety, arousal, stress or activation. Though these concepts are not synonymous, their relationships to the performance have sufficient similarities to lump them together for the present purposes. Anxiety denotes worry or emotional tension, arousal denotes a continuum from sleep to high excitement, stress implies an agent that induces strain in the organism and activation refers to the metabolic state in the 'fight or flight' reaction. Irrespective of which concept is adopted the effects of the biological responses on performance are generally assumed to fit an inverted U curve. A moderate level of 'anxiety' about the forthcoming activity is desirable to induce the right levels of motivation for action. The simpler the task the higher will be the level of anxiety that can be tolerated before performance efficiency begins to fall (Figure 5.1).

Although the inverted U model is somewhat simplistic, it does illustrate that over-anxiety has a detrimental effect on the physical and psychomotor elements that comprise sports performance. In such instances anxiety-reducing strategies will have an ergogenic effect. The

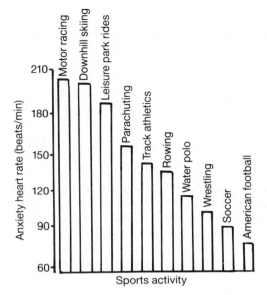

Figure 5.2 Pre-activity heart rate for various sports and recreations.

athlete or mentor may have to choose between mental relaxation techniques or drugs to alleviate anxiety.

There are various indices which the behavioural scientist employs in measuring anxiety in field conditions such as sport, especially pre-competition. These include hand tremor, restlessness or other subjective estimates of 'tension', paper and pencil tests and so on. Linked to these are physiological indices which demonstrate increased sympathetic tone. These include muscular tension as measured by electromyography, galvanic skin response or skin conductance and elevated concentrations of stress hormones or their metabolites in blood or in urine. These may be important to consider if the mechanisms by which the ergogenic or adverse effects of anxiety-reducing drugs operate are to be understood.

Although high levels of anxiety generally militate against performance and so favour attempts to reduce anxiety, the anxiety level depends very much on the nature of the sport as well as on the individual concerned. Generally, high anxiety is associated with brief and high-risk activities. A league table of anxiety responses pre-start (Figure 5.2) as reflected in the emotional tachycardia shows motor-racing, ski-jumping and downhill skiing to be top of the list. Activities like parachuting and high acceleration rides in leisure parks induce strong anxiety reactions. In these cases the heart rates have been found to correlate highly with adrenaline levels in blood and in urine (Reilly *et al.*, 1985). American football is lowest in the table, possibly because of the practice of meditation and relaxation techniques and the long duration of such games.

Professional athletes regularly subjected to situations of high psychological stress tend to adapt and at this elite level highly anxious personalities are rare. The anxiety reaction of professional soccer players, for example, is highly reproducible although there are noticeable trends. Heart rates in the dressing room tend to be higher when playing at home rather than away, because players are subject to more critical scrutiny by a home audience. Anxiety is highest in goalkeepers, for whose mistakes the team is usually punished severely. Players returning to the team after a spell of injury or making an initial appearance in the premier team show higher heart rates than their normal pre-match values. It is hardly surprising to find that goalkeepers are the most vulnerable members of the team to stress-related illnesses such as stomach ulcers.

Attenuation of over-anxiety may be important in games players for reasons of safety. Anxiety has been found to correlate with joint and muscle injuries in soccer, the more anxious players tending to get injured most often. This supports the notion of injury proneness: the mechanism is probably lack of commitment or hesitancy in critical events that might promote injury, such as tackling (Sanderson, 1981). Some soccer players are in the habit of taking a nip of whisky immediately prior to going onto the pitch, the communal bottle being euphemistically referred to as 'team spirit'. The inhibiting effects of alcohol are exploited by tournament rugby players, who are not averse to drinking beer in between rounds of 'rugby sevens' competitions, for example.

Obviously there is a thin line to tread between on the one hand reducing anxiety to enhance well-being and mental states prior to competing in sport and on the other hand impairing performance because of a disruption in motor co-ordination accompanying the treatment. The outcome depends on the concentrations of the drug, the timing of ingestion and the individual susceptibility to it. There are also possibilities of adaptation to chronic use of the drug and of a drug dependence developing. Residual effects may carry over to the days that follow, affecting training or subsequent competitive performance. These aspects are now considered in the context of alcohol in sports and exercise.

5.3 Alcohol

The alcohols are a group of chemicals, most of which are toxic. The most common is ethanol or ethyl alcohol which is obtained by the fermentation of sugar. It is non-toxic except in large and chronic doses and has been enjoyed as a beverage for many centuries.

Ethyl alcohol is both a drug and a food, accounting for about 100 kcal (420 kJ) per adult of the UK population each day. Its energy value per unit weight (kcal/g), the Atwater factor, is 7 compared with a value of 9 for fat but this is higher than the value of 4 for both carbohydrate and protein. Wine contains about 10% alcohol and so a 1 litre bottle will have about 100 g with a caloric content of 705 kcal (2951 kJ). The value of alcohol as a foodstuff is limited as it is metabolized mainly in the liver and at a fixed rate of about 100 mg/kg body weight/hour. For a 70 kg individual this amounts to 7 g alcohol hourly. The energy is not available to active skeletal muscle and consequently it is not possible to exercise oneself to sobriety. Beer contains some electrolytes but its subsequent diuretic effect makes it less than the ideal agent of rehydration after hard physical training.

Alcohol is a polar substance which is freely miscible in water. This is due to the fact that alcohol molecules are held together by the same sort of intermolecular forces as water, namely hydrogen bonds. The alcohol molecule is also soluble in fat, it is small and has a weak charge. (As the lipophilic alkyl group becomes larger and the hydrophilic group smaller, the alcohol molecules associate preferentially with other alcohol, hydrocarbon or lipid molecules rather than water.) It easily penetrates biological membranes and can be absorbed unaltered from the stomach and more quickly from the small intestine. The rate of absorption is influenced by the amount of food in the stomach, whether there are gas molecules in the drink and the concentration of alcohol in the drink. Absorption is quickest if alcohol is drunk on an empty stomach, if gas molecules are present in the drink and the alcohol content is high. Intense mental concentration, lowered body temperature or physical exertion tend to slow the rate of absorption.

From the gastrointestinal tract the alcohol is transported to the liver by means of the hepatic circulation. The activity of the enzyme alcohol dehydrogenase, present chiefly in the liver, governs the disappearance of alcohol from the body. In the liver, alcohol dehydrogenase converts the alcohol to acetaldehyde and it is then converted to acetic acid or acetate by aldehyde dehydrogenase. About 75% of the alcohol taken up by the blood is released as acetate into the circulation. The acetate is then oxidized to CO_2 and water within the Krebs (or citric acid) cycle. An alternative metabolic route for acetate is its activation to acetyl coenzyme A and further reactions to form fatty acids, ketone bodies, amino acids and steroids.

Ethyl alcohol is distributed throughout the body via the circulatory system and enters all the body water pools and tissues, including the central nervous system. Its distribution among the body fluids and tissues depends on several factors such as blood flow, mass and permeability of the tissue. Organs such as the brain, lungs, liver and kidneys reach equilibrium quickly while skeletal muscle with its relatively poorer blood supply attains its peak alcohol concentration more slowly. Initially, alcohol moves rapidly from blood into the tissues. When absorption is complete, arterial alcohol concentration falls and alcohol diffuses from the tissues into the capillary bed. This means that alcohol concentrations remain high in the peripheral venous blood due to the slower rates of metabolism and excretion.

The metabolism of alcohol in the liver is unaffected by its concentration in the blood. Some alcohol is eliminated in the breath, but this is usually less than 5% of the total amount metabolized. This route is utilized in assessing safe levels for driving, forming the basis of the breathalyser tests. Small amounts of alcohol are also excreted in urine and in sweat if exercise is performed while drunk. Higher excretion rates through the lungs, urine and sweat are produced at high environmental temperatures and at high blood alcohol levels.

With a single drink the blood alcohol level usually peaks about 45 minutes after ingestion. This is the point where any influence on performance will be most evident. Effect on performance will generally be greater on the ascending limb than for a corresponding value on the descending limb of the blood alcohol curve; the rate of change and the direction of change of the blood alcohol concentration are more crucial factors than is the length of time alcohol is in the bloodstream. The peak is delayed about 15 minutes if strenuous exercise precedes the ingestion. This may be due to the reduction in blood flow to the gut that accompanies exercise, the increased blood flow to skeletal muscle and the needs of the thermoregulatory system post-exercise.

Besides the exogenous ethanol in body fluids, trace amounts of ethanol are synthesized endogenously. This endogenous ethanol is thought to arise both from bacterial fermentation in the gut and from action of alcohol dehydrogenase on acetaldehyde derived from pyruvate. Blood levels of endogenous alcohol in man are very low, ranging only up to about 7.5 mg in total.

Studies on alcohol and exercise are notoriously difficult to control, as most subjects will recognize the taste of the experimental treatment. Most experimentors use vodka in orange juice as the alcohol beverage: the placebo can include enough vodka to taste but not enough to produce a measurable blood alcohol concentration. Another strategy is to put a noseclip on the subject who is then given anaesthetic throat lozenges. Subjects vary in their responses to alcohol as does the same subject from day to day, making inferences from laboratory studies difficult. As the effects of alcohol differ with body size, dosage is usually administered according to differences in body weight. Effects also vary with the level of blood alcohol induced but there is not general international agreement on acceptable maximum levels for day to day activities such as driving. Alcohol doses that render subjects 'legless' have little practical relevance in exercise studies and so experimental levels are usually low to moderate.

5.3.1 ACTION OF ALCOHOL ON THE NERVOUS SYSTEM

The effects of ethanol administration on central nervous tissue are due to direct action rather than to acetaldehyde, its first breakdown product. Following ethanol ingestion very little acetaldehyde crosses the blood–brain barrier, despite elevated levels in the blood. Alcohol has a general effect on neural transmission by influencing axonal membranes and slowing nerve conductance. The permeability of the axonal membrane to potassium and sodium is altered by the lowering of central calcium levels that results from ingesting alcohol (Wesnes and Warburton, 1983). Alcohol has differential effects on the central neurotransmitters, acetylcholine, serotonin, noradrenaline and dopamine.

Alcohol blocks the release of acetylcholine and disrupts its synthesis. As a result transmission in the central cholinergic pathways will be lowered. The ascending reticular cholinergic pathway determines the level of cortical arousal and the flow of sensory information to be evaluated by the cortex. The lowering of electrocortical arousal reduces the awareness of stressful information and the ability of the individual to attend to specific stimuli. These de-arousing changes are reflected in alterations in the electroencephalogram with moderate to large doses of alcohol. The obvious results are impairments in concentration, attention, simple and complex reaction times, skilled performance and eventually short-term memory, balance and speech.

Alcohol decreases serotonin turnover in the central nervous system by inhibiting tryptophan hydroxylase, the enzyme essential for its biosynthesis. Activity in the neurones of serotonergic pathways in important for the experience of anxiety; output of corticosteroid hormones from the adrenal cortex increases the activity in these neurones. Alcohol has an opposing action and so may reduce the tension that is felt by the individual in a stressful situation.

An effect of alcohol is to increase activity in central noradrenergic pathways. This is transient and is followed, some hours later, by a decrease in activity. Catecholaminergic pathways are implicated in the control of mood states, activation of these pathways promoting happy and merry states. The fall in noradrenaline turnover as the blood concentrations drop ties in with the reversal of mood that follows the initial drunken euphoric state. This is exacerbated by large doses of alcohol as these tend to give rise to depression.

Alcohol also has an effect on cerebral energy metabolism: the drug decreases glucose utilization in the brain. As glucose is the main substrate furnishing energy for nerve cells, the result is that the lowered glucose level may induce mental fatigue. This will be reflected in failing cognitive functions, decline in concentration and in information processing. It is unlikely that exercise, *per se*, will offset these effects.

The disruption of acetylcholine synthesis and release means that alcohol acts as a depressant, exerting its effect on the reticular activating system, whose activity represents the level of physiological arousal. It also has a depressant effect on the cortex: it first affects the frontal centres of the cortex before affecting the cerebellum. In large quantities it will affect speech and muscular co-ordination, eventually inducing sedation. In smaller doses it inhibits cerebral control mechanisms, freeing the brain from its normal inhibition. This release of inhibition has been blamed for aggressive and violent conduct of individuals behaving out of character when under the influence of alcohol. Undoubtedly alcohol has been a factor in crowd violence and football

Table 5.1 Demonstrable effects of alcohol at different blood alcohol concentrations

Concentration level (mg/100 ml blood)	Effects
32	Enhanced sense of well-being; retarded simple reaction time; impaired hand-eye co-ordination
64	Mild loss of social inhibition; impaired judgement
80	Marked loss of social inhibition; co-ordination reduced; noticeably 'under the influence'
112	Apparent clumsiness; loss of physical control; tendency towards extreme responses; definite drunkeness is noted

hooliganism on the terraces. This belief has led to the banning of alcohol at football grounds in Scotland, severe restriction of alcohol sales at English League grounds following the crowd control problems at the European Cup final in Brussels in 1985 and restriction of alcohol at cricket grounds in England after riots at an England – Pakistan match in 1987.

Clearly, alcohol will have deleterious effects on performance in sports that require fast reactions, complex decision making and highly skilled actions. It will also have an impact on hand–eye co-ordination, on tracking tasks such as driving and on vigilance tasks such as long-distance sailing. An effect on tracking tasks is that control movements lose their normal smoothness and precision and become more abrupt or jerky. In vigilance tasks, some studies show a deterioration in perform-ance with time on task (Tong, Henderson and Chipperfield, 1980). At high doses of alcohol, meaningful sport becomes impractical or downright dangerous. Progressive effects of alcohol at different blood alcohol concentrations are summarized in Table 5.1. An important effect of alcohol, not listed, is that it diminishes the ability to process appreciable amounts of information arriving simultaneously from two different sources.

The most frequently cited study of alcohol facilitating human performance was the classical experiment of Ikai and Steinhaus (1961). They showed that in some cases moderate alcohol doses could improve isometric muscular strength. This result was similar to that obtained by cheering and loud vocal encouragement. They explained the effect on the basis of central inhibition of the impulse traffic in the nerve fibres of the skeletal muscles during maximal effort. This depression of the inhibitory effect of certain centres in the central nervous system may allow routine practices to proceed normally without any disturbing effects. It should be noted that this finding has not generally been replicated when other aspects of muscular performance are considered. These are reviewed in a later section.

5.3.2 ALCOHOL AND HEALTH

The effects of alcohol on health are usually viewed in terms of chronic alcoholism. Persistent drinking leads to a dependence on alcohol so that it becomes addictive. Most physicians emphasize that alcoholism is a disease rather than a vice and devise therapy accordingly. The result of excessive drinking is ultimately manifested in liver disease: cirrhosis, a serious hardening and degeneration of liver tissue, is fatal for many heavy drinkers. Cancer is also more likely to develop in a cirrhotic liver. Cardiomyopathy or damage to the heart muscle can also result from years of hard drinking. Other pathological conditions associated with alcohol abuse include generalized skeletal myopathy and cancers of pharynx and larynx. Impairment of brain function also occurs, alcoholic psychoses being a common cause of hospitalization in psychiatric wards.

Alcohol was formerly used as an anaesthetic until it was realized that it was too dangerous to supply in large quantities for that purpose. The result of applying alcohol to living cells is that the protoplasm of the cells precipitates as a consequence of dehydration. Long-term damage to tissue in the central nervous system may be an unwanted outcome of habitual heavy drinking.

Heavy drinking is not compatible with serious athletics. For the athlete, drinking is usually done only in moderation, an infrequent respite from the ascetic regimens of physical training, though the odd end-of-season binge is customary. Nevertheless drinking is a social convention in many sports, such as rugby, squash and water-polo. The sensible athlete drinks moderately and occasionally, avoiding alcohol for at least 24 hours before competing. Hangovers may persist for a day and disturb concentration in sports involving complex skills. The attitude of the retired athlete may be very different. If his active career is terminated abruptly and the free time that retirement releases is taken up by social drinking, the result may well be a gradual deterioration in physical condition with body weight increasing and fitness declining. In this context the effect of alcohol on the ex-athlete will be quite harmful. The case of the great Kenyan distance runner Henry Rono is a salutory example. Six years after setting world records at 3000 m, 3000 m steeplechase, 5000 m and 10 000 m, he was referred for treatment to a rehabilitation clinic for chronic alcoholics.

Various institutions within sports medicine have addressed the problems of alcohol and exercise. In 1982 the American College of Sports Medicine set out a position statement on alcohol which was unequivocally against any indulgence. It underlined the adverse effects of alcohol on health and condemned the resort to alcohol by athletes. Its estimate was that there were 10 million adult problem drinkers in the United States and an additional 3.3 million in its 14–17 years age range. Any evidence of beneficial aspects of alcohol was dismissed without mention.

There is a belief that moderate drinking has some positive benefits for health. Small amounts increase the flow of gastric juices and thereby stimulate digestion: in large doses alcohol irritates the stomach lining, causing gastritis and even vomiting of blood. A national survey of lifestyles in England and Wales provided support for the view that healthy people tended to drink a little. Among men under 60, the likelihood of high blood pressure was found to increase with the amount of alcohol consumed. For older men and for women, light drinking was associated with lower blood pressure, even when effects due to body weight were taken into account (Stepney, 1987).

It is thought also that moderate drinking provides a degree of protection against coronary heart disease. This may have been nurtured in the vineyards of France where a habitually modest consumption of wine is associated with a low incidence of heart disease. One report claimed that myocardial infarction rates were lower in moderate drinkers than in non-drinkers (Willett *et al.*, 1980). A possible mechanism is the reduction in hypertension and the relaxation from business cares that drinking can bring. A link has been shown by an increase in high-density lipoprotein cholesterol levels with moderate levels of drinking alcohol. High-density lipoprotein particles remove cholesterol from the tissues and transfer it into other particles in the blood; low-density lipoprotein on the other hand, obtains its cholesterol from these other particles and transfers it to the tissues. A high ratio of high-density to low-density lipoprotein fractions is generally found in well-trained endurance athletes, a low ratio being indicative of poor coronary health. The mechanism by which alcohol would raise the high-density lipoprotein cholesterol has not been fully explained.

It seems that for a healthy athlete in a good state of training, occasional drinking of alcohol in moderation will have little adverse effect. It is important to emphasize that any such occasional bouts of drinking should be restrained and should follow rather than precede training sessions, whose training stimulus is likely to be lowered by the soporific influence of drinking alcohol before strenuous exertion.

5.3.3 ALCOHOL AND PHYSIOLOGICAL RESPONSES TO EXERCISE

Alcohol ingestion has been shown to lower muscle glycogen at rest compared with control conditions. As pre-start glycogen levels are important for sustained exercise at an intensity of about 70–80% $\dot{V}O_2$ max., such as marathon running, taking alcohol in the 24 hours before such endurance activities is ill-advised. Effects of alcohol on the metabolic responses to sub-maximal exercise seem to be small. Juhlin-Dannfelt and co-workers (1977) reported that alcohol does not impair lipolysis or free fatty acid utilization during exercise. It may decrease splanchnic glucose output, decrease the potential contribution of energy from liver gluconeogenesis, cause a more pronounced decline in blood glucose levels and decrease the leg muscle uptake of glucose towards the end of a 3-hour run.

Some studies have shown an increase in oxygen uptake ($\dot{V}O_2$) at a fixed sub-maximal exercise intensity after alcohol ingestion. This may be due to a poorer co-ordination of the active muscles as the decrease in mechanical efficiency, implied by the elevation in $\dot{V}O_2$, is not a consistent finding. Related to this is an increase in blood lactate levels with alcohol; metabolism of ethanol shunts lactate away from the gluconeogenic pathway and leads to an increase in the ratio of lactate to pyruvate. It is possible that elevated blood lactate concentrations during exercise, after taking alcohol, may reflect impairment in clearance of lactate rather than an increase in production by the exercising muscles. A failure to clear lactate would militate against performance of strenuous exercise.

Alcohol does not seem to have adverse effects on $\dot{V}O_2$ max. or on metabolic responses to high intensity exercise approaching $\dot{V}O_2$ max. levels. At high doses (up to 200 mg%, i.e. 0.20% blood alcohol level) it is understandable that athletes may feel disinclined towards maximal efforts that elicit $\dot{V}O_2$ max. values and a reduction in peak $\dot{V}E$ is usually observed (Blomqvist, Saltin and Mitchell, 1970). Similarly, they may be poorly motivated to sustain high intensity exercise for as long as they would normally do.

Although alcohol has not conclusively been shown to alter $\dot{V}E$, stroke volume, or muscle blood flow at sub-maximal exercise levels, peripheral vascular resistance is decreased. This is because of the vasodilatory effect of alcohol on the peripheral blood vessels. This would increase heat loss from the surface of the skin and cause a drop in body temperature. This would be dangerous if alcohol is taken in conjunction with exercise in cold conditions. Sampling from a hip-flask of whisky on the ski slopes may bring an immediate inner glow and feeling of warmth but its disturbance of normal thermoregulation may put the recreational skier at risk of hypothermia. Frost-bitten mountaineers especially should avoid drinking alcohol as the peripheral vasodilation it induces would cause the body temperature to fall further. In hot conditions, alcohol is also inadvisable as it acts as a diuretic and would exacerbate problems of dehydration.

Studies of maximum muscular strength, in the main, find no influence of moderate to medium doses of alcohol on maximum isometric tension. Similar results apply to dynamic functions, such as peak torque measured on isokinetic dynamometers. Muscular endurance is generally assessed by requiring the subject to hold a fixed percentage of maximum for as long as possible. Here, too, the influences of moderate alcohol doses are generally found to be non-significant. This may be because the tests represent gross aspects of muscular function and as such are insensitive to the effects of the drug.

5.3.4 ALCOHOL IN AIMING SPORTS

In aiming sports, a steady limb is needed to provide a firm platform for launching the missile at its target or to keep the weapon still. Examples of such sports are archery, billiards, darts, pistol shooting and snooker. There are also aiming components in sports such as fencing and modern pentathlon, especially in the rifle shooting discipline of the latter. In some of these sports alcohol levels are now officially monitored, while in others, notably darts, drinking is a conventional complement of the sport itself.

The Grand National Archery Society in the UK has not yet banned the use of alcohol in its competitions and so alcohol is taken in small doses in the belief that it relaxes the archer, thereby steadying the hand as well as the nerve. In order to avoid fluctuating blood alcohol concentrations the archer, like the dart thrower, tries to keep topping up the levels to prevent them from falling down the descending limb of the curve.

To understand how alcohol might affect the archer it is useful to look at the task *in toto*. The competitive player has to shoot three dozen arrows at each of four targets – 90, 70, 60 and 50 m away – to complete an FITA (the world governing body) round. The highest possible score is 1440, 10 points being the maximum for each perfect shot. The world record score is 1342 achieved by 1984 Olympic Games champion Darrel Pace back in 1979. Technological improvements in bow design have helped to produce such outstanding scores, leaving the gap to perfection due to human factors. The modern bow has two slot-in limbs which insert into a magnesium handle section and stabilizers which help to minimize vibration and turning of the bow. Muscle strength is needed to draw the bow while muscle endurance is called for to hold it steady, usually for about 8 s for each shot, while the sight is aligned with the target. Deflection of the arrow tip by 0.02 mm at 90 m causes the arrow to miss the target, which gives some idea of the hand steadiness required. The archer, before release or loose, pulls the arrow towards and through the clicker (a blade on the side of the bow which aids in measuring draw length). He reacts to the sound of the clicker hitting the side of the bow handle by releasing the string which in effect shoots the arrow. Archers are coached to react to the clicker by allowing the muscles to relax; a slow reaction to the clicker is generally recognized as hesitation. This affects the smoothness of the loose and is reflected in muscle tremor causing a 'snatched loose'. For these reasons, the effects of alcohol on reaction time, arm steadiness, muscle strength and endurance, and the electromyogram of one of the arm muscles were selected as appropriate parameters to isolate and study under experimental conditions (Reilly and Halliday, 1985).

In the experiment, nine subjects underwent a battery of tests under four conditions: sober, placebo, 0.02% blood alcohol level and 0.05% blood alcohol level. The alcohol doses were administered in three equal

Table 5.2 Effects of the alcohol treatments on four experimental tests (mean ± s.d.) (from Reilly and Halliday, 1985)

Variables	Sober	Placebo	0.02% BAC	0.05% BAC
Arm steadiness:				
time off-target (s)	2.64 ± 0.89	3.05 ± 0.74	3.24 ± 1.01	8.17 ± 1.49
Isometric strength (kg)	55.4 ± 4.9	56.8 ± 3.8	54.9 ± 5.7	53.0 ± 7.9
Muscular endurance (s)	11.4 ± 2.1	12.0 ± 2.5	12.0 ± 2.0	10.8 ± 2.0
Reaction time (ms)	211 ± 6.5	209 ± 8.5	223 ± 9.6	226 ± 11.2

volumes to total 500 ml over 15 minutes, 45 minutes being allowed for peak blood alcohol levels to be attained. The doses to elicit the desirable blood alcohol levels were calculated according to the formula of Hicks (1976) which was shown to be effective:

$$A = \frac{(454)\,(W)\,(R)\,(BAC + 0.0002)}{(0.8)\,(0.95)}$$

where A = ml 95% ethanol
     W = body weight (lb)
     R = distribution coefficient of 0.765
     BAC = desired blood alcohol concentration (0.05% = 0.0005)

A summary of the results for the performance measurement appears in Table 5.2. There was no effect of alcohol on the muscular strength and muscular endurance measures; the holding time in the endurance test was about the same time as the archer normally holds the bow drawn before shooting, so that this test turned out to be reasonably realistic. Reaction time was significantly slowed by the lower alcohol dose, a further small delay occurring at the higher blood alcohol level. The more sensitive response of auditory reaction time to alcohol would mean, in practice, a slower reaction to the clicker and a faulty loose. Another adverse effect noted was the impairment in steadiness of the extended arm. Performance was degraded, especially at the 0.05% blood alcohol level, and the variability in arm steadiness also increased with alcohol. This effect contradicts the conventional wisdom in archery and may have been due to the high load on the arm muscles when holding the bow drawn. It is possible also that alcohol only operates to advantage in steadying the limb in contexts more competitive than laboratory experiments.

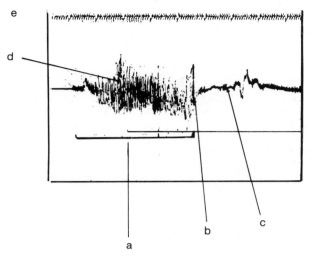

Figure 5.3 The electromyographic profile of an arm muscle while holding the bow drawn: (a) holding time; (b) the point of loose; (c) post-loose muscular activity; (d) tremor; (e) the time scale of events marked in 100 ms.

Some benefits were noted in the electromyographic profile (Figure 5.3). A clearer loose was observed at the low alcohol levels which would be valuable in promoting a smoother release. This was supplemented by a tendency towards a reduced tremor in the muscle with both alcohol treatments. Together, these effects would indicate greater muscle relaxation, the tremor being normally associated with a snatched loose. These factors were partly offset by the longer holding time prior to loose induced by the alcohol treatments. The overall conclusion was that alcohol has differential effects on tasks related to archery, depending on the concentrations, the components of the performance analysed and individual reactivity to the drug.

The deleterious effects of alcohol on some aspects of archery would not apply to other aiming sports such as darts and pistol shooting. In these the loading on the arm muscles is light, so a greater arm steadiness is likely to be induced by the drug. Another consideration is that the timing of the release is at the discretion of the subject and so is unaffected by a retarded reaction time. Reactions will have importance where the target is moving: it is noteworthy that the discipline of clay-pigeon shooting, for example, is not steeped in a history of alcohol use.

The bar-room sports such as snooker, billiards and darts have the alcohol industry as an adjunct to their matches. At the highest level of competition these sports are a popular television spectacle. Although it is widely thought that the top performers swig large quantities of alcohol, this is not the case. Imbibition is regular but in small doses so that a moderate blood alcohol level is continually maintained (Needless to say, at high blood alcohol levels, 0.15% or more, whole-body stability and mental concentration would be degraded and any possible ergogenic effect would be swamped.) Alcohol is not prohibited in these sports though other drugs are.

In those sports that discourage alcohol for competition there is a disharmony in standards for what constitutes legality. (Alcohol is banned in several sports, for example modern pentathlon, fencing and shooting.) It is worthy of note that the legal limit for driving differs between countries: in Norway the limit is 50 mg/100 ml, in Denmark it is twice that level while in the UK the safety limit is intermediate at 80 mg/100 ml. These values refer to alcohol in blood: the corresponding levels for breath and for urine are 35 μg/100 ml and 107 mg/100 ml respectively. The Amateur Fencing Association in Britain has adopted the Norwegian value as its limit for competition and has incorporated dope testing at its contests since 1984. At the request of the international governing body for fencing, alcohol tests are now carried out at the Olympic Games, although it is generally accepted that alcohol abuse is not a major problem in this sport.

Drug testing for alcohol is a two-stage process (Beckett and Cowan, 1979). A breath sample is analysed immediately after competition using a standard breathalyser. If the result indicates a level greater than 50 mg/100 ml a blood sample is obtained. This is analysed by gas chromatography which is more sensitive than the breath test. It is possible to obtain accurate and reliable results with a spectrophotometer.

Testing for alcohol is also performed on competitors in the shooting event of the modern pentathlon. Here participants are disadvantaged by losing time in settling down to prepare for taking their shots. Recovering from their prior activity is important if the shots are to be on target. Although alcohol might help competitors to relax while taking aim, it has little ergogenic benefits in the other disciplines of the pentathlon. For various reasons, tranquillisers and beta-blocking agents have been preferred. These are considered in the sections that follow.

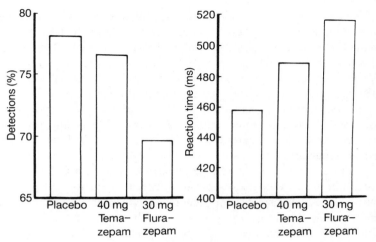

Figure 5.4 The effects of temazepam (40 mg) and flurazepam (30 mg) on the percentage of correct detections and the reaction time in a rapid information-processing task. The tasks were performed the morning after nightly administration of the drugs. (From Wesnes and Warburton, 1983: reprinted with permission of John Wiley and Sons Ltd.)

5.4 Benzodiazepines

Benzodiazepines, derivatives of benzodiazepine, are widely employed as tranquillisers in the population at large and have been used for calming or sedative purposes in sports. They are included in the list of drugs that may be taken by sportsmen. There are now over two dozen benzodiaze-pine drugs and these form over 90% of the tranquilliser market. More than 20 doses of these drugs per head of the USA population are prescribed annually, giving an idea of the vast scale of consumption.

The first benzodiazepine drug was synthesized in the mid-1950s, the best known of those that followed being Librium (chlordiazepoxide hydrochloride) introduced in the USA in 1960 and Valium (diazepam) in 1963. The benzodiazepines have systematically replaced the bar-biturates and the propranediol derivatives as drugs of clinical choice in treating stress and anxiety. There is little evidence that the barbiturates had a major use among active athletes as an ergogenic aid in the years when they were being widely prescribed, although they may have been used in more recent years.

Benzodiazepines decrease stress response indices such as skin conductance and plasma corticosterone levels. They have been found to reduce anxiety in psychiatric and non-psychiatric patients and have demonstrated a superiority over barbiturates in clinical conditions. The drugs affect various neurotransmitters, the cholinergic and serotonergic effects having importance in reducing the stress response.

The benzodiazepines decrease the turnover in hemispheric cholinergic neurones by blocking the release of acetylcholine. By thus lowering the activity in cholinergic pathways, the drugs should have an adverse effect on human performance. Deterioration in the detection of sensory signals and in reaction time in a rapid information-processing task with nightly doses of flurazapam and temazapam have been found the morning after taking the drugs (Figure 5.4). The carry-over effect is due to the long half-lives of these particular drugs. Other types of performance affected include the rate of tapping, motor manipulation and complex co-ordination tasks, as well as real and simulated driving.

The function of one particular cholinergic pathway is to trigger the release of corticotrophic releasing factor (CRF) from the hypothalamus into the pituitary blood vessels and produce a spurt of adrenocorticotrophic hormone (ACTH) from the anterior pituitary. The benzodiazepines would lower the emission of corticosteroid hormones from the adrenal cortex by affecting ACTH release as a result of blocking cholinergic activity.

The benzodiazepines have been found to decelerate the turnover of noradrenaline. This effect is more apparent in conditions where the noradrenaline levels have been increased by stress. This change is not the basis of the drug's anti-anxiety action as repeated dosing with oxazepam results in a rapid tolerance to the decrease in noradrenaline turnover, whilst the drug maintains its anti-anxiety properties (Wesnes and Warburton, 1983). Similarly, dopamine turnover is retarded by benzodiazepines but this effect is unrelated to the drugs' anti-anxiety properties.

The main anti-anxiety action of the benzodiazepines seems to stem from the reduction in serotonergic activity which the drugs produce. Serotonergic neurones are important in the experience of anxiety so that this feeling is attenuated by the drugs. The effects of the benzodiazepines on serotonergic neurones may be mediated by a primary action of the drugs on gamma aminobutyric acid (GABA). (It is thought that administration of GABA has been tried by some sports competitors.) The GABA-releasing neurones are primarily inhibitory and it is possible that when these are stimulated by the benzodiazepines the release of serotonin is inhibited. The GABA system is recognized as playing a crucial role in anxiety: some anxiety-related states may be due to diminished transmission at the level of GABA receptors which are functionally linked to benzodiazepine recognition sites (Corda, Concas and Biggio, 1986).

The effects of benzodiazepines on components of human performance will depend on the dosage and on the particular drugs. Oxazepam, diazepam, nitrazepam, flurazepam, chlordiazepoxide are all 1,4 derivatives. Clobazam, a 1,5 benzodiazepine derivative, does not seem to impair psychomotor performance but does retain its anti-anxiety properties (Wesnes and Warburton, 1983) and so may have more applications than the others in sport and exercise contexts.

Following the bans on alcohol overuse in the modern pentathlon, athletes at the 1972 Olympic Games in Munich were found to have used benzodiazepines and other tranquillisers, such as meprobamate, as anti-anxiety agents. These were thought preferable to alcohol as they might reduce anxiety without the potential adverse effects on judgement and co-ordination associated with alcohol. Meprobamate acts as a mild tranquilliser without producing drowsiness. It is highly addictive and reduces tolerance to alcohol. The benzodiazepines are relatively safe in that they have low toxicity and few side effects. They can induce a dependence in chronic users and severe withdrawal symptoms are experienced when patients are taken off them abruptly.

One of the primary effects of the GABA-mediated reaction to benzodiazepines is that the drugs act as muscle relaxants. For this reason, they can be beneficial in aiding recovery from spastic type muscle injuries. The effect is associated with a feeling of freedom from 'nerves' and tension. The repercussions for muscle function in extreme exertion have not been systematically explored. Spontaneous activity of animals is reduced under the influence of these drugs. A preliminary study of two benzodiazepines (Cabri, et al., Vrije Universiteit, Brussels, personal communication, 1987) suggested that the effects were dependent on the type of contraction, its velocity, the particular drug and the individual susceptibility. Beneficial effects were apparent in concentric contractions of the quadriceps, the muscle group examined. Adverse effects were more pronounced during fast velocities of contraction and during eccentric work. Although it is interesting to speculate on how the drugs affect the cross-bridging of actin and myosin under these conditions, the precise mechanism involved in their effects on muscle function remains to be explained.

The effects of benzodiazepines on sustained exercise performance are similarly poorly documented. In resting normal humans, coronary blood flow is increased by 22.5% by diazepam but more so (73%) in persons with coronary artery disease. Whether the drugs benefit the angina of effort is unknown (Powles, 1981).

Barbiturates and sedatives have long been used in sleeping pills. Such a use, to facilitate the sleep of athletes the night before competition, is likely to be counterproductive because of a residual de-arousing effect the following day.

The 'hangover' effect of benzodiazepines was found to be greater for flurazepam (30 mg) than for temazepam (40 mg); although the former produced better sleep, it resulted in lowered clearheadedness on waking and impaired performance on a rapid visual information processing task (Wesnes and Warburton, 1984).

The 'hangover' effect of sleeping tablets, including benzodiazepines, is likely to disturb complex skills more than simple motor tasks performed early the following day; depending on the sport, an increase in errors may promote a higher risk of injury. Similarly, the prescription of sleeping pills to assist adaptation to time-zone changes is likely to have limited success in combating jet-lag symptoms. Use of behavioural methods of adaptation is more productive, while orally ingested melatonin may be a practical method of countering jet lag in the future. Low doses of benzodiazepines may benefit shift workers who have difficulty in sleeping during the day after a nocturnal shift. A study of simulated shift work by Wesnes and Warburton (1986) found that 10–20 mg doses of temazepam helped daytime sleep without detrimental residual effects on subsequent information processing.

The circadian or 24-hour rhythm in arousal may have implications for the pharmacological effects of anti-anxiety drugs. The optimum dosage of drugs affecting the nervous system differs with the time of day at which they are administered. The barbiturate dose that is safe in the evening may have exaggerated effects in early morning (Luce, 1973). The same is true for alcohol and this is reflected in social drinking habits: usually only alcoholics drink before breakfast and in the late morning. The diurnal variation in responses to benzodiazepines and the implications this has on the dosage at different times of day for effective pre-contest tranquillization does not seem to have been the subject of any serious research attention.

5.5 Marijuana

Marijuana is obtained from the hemp plant *Cannabis sativa*. It contains the compound tetrahydrocannabinol which accounts for its phsychological effects. These include a sedating and euphoric feeling of well-being and relaxation, with a sensation of sleepiness. Balance may be disturbed; aggression and motivation to perform may be blunted. Maximum muscular strength is reduced, probably because of the reduced drive towards all-out efforts.

Largely because of its promotion of happy and euphoric mood states, marijuana has been prominent among the drugs of abuse, notably by youngsters and college students in the USA and Europe. A report of the US Department of Health and Human Services, *Student Drug Use in America 1975 to 1980*, claimed that nearly one-third of students had tried marijuana before entering high school. This background of experience with the drug might explain its popularity among young athletes as a mode of release from tension during the competitive season.

Persistent marijuana smoking is incompatible with serious athletic training. The single-mindedness of the athlete will be disturbed by the demotivating influence of the drug. A few cigarettes of marijuana may cause minor changes in personality while high doses can induce hallucinations, delusions and psychotic-like symptoms. The major abuse of marijuana has been by collegiate games teams, playing basketball and football, in the USA. The practice of smoking marijuana is generally condemned by athletic trainers and coaches in that country.

5.6 Nicotine

The tobacco leaf, *Nicotiana tabacum*, is the source of the cigarettes on which the massive tobacco industry is based. As the tobacco burns it generates about 4000 different compounds, including carbon monoxide, ammonia, hydrogen cyanide, many carcinogens, DDT and tar. Carbon monoxide (CO) reduces the oxygen transport capacity of the blood by combining with haemoglobin (Hb) and so takes the place of oxygen in the bloodstream, adversely affecting aerobic exercise performance. The affinity of CO for haemoglobin is 230 times that of oxygen. Tobacco smoke contains about 4% CO; smoking 10-12 cigarettes a day results in a blood COHb level of 4.9%, 15–25 a day raises the value to 6.3% while 30–40 each day takes the level to 9.3%. Adverse effects are noticeable only during physical exertion and after smoking it may take 24 hours or more for blood CO levels to return to normal. The smoke also paralyses the cilia in the respiratory passages so that their filtering becomes ineffective and the individual is more susceptible to respiratory tract infections.

The anti-smoking argument is centred around the links between smoking and cancer. Another strong link has been shown between smoking and hardening of the peripheral arteries and deterioration of the circulation to the limbs. Other long-term health hazards associated with heavy smoking are acceleration of coronary atherosclerosis, pulmonary emphysema and cerebral vascular disease.

About 30% of the adult population throughout the world smoke cigarettes and it is likely that double this number have sampled cigarettes at one time or another. As passive inhalation of smoke by non-users of tobacco – especially in crowded public places – has similar effects to those in smokers, smoking in public facilities is now restricted in many countries. About 20% of the smoke exhaled can be re-circulated in passive inhalation.

The psychological and addictive effects of smoking are attributable to nicotine. Smokers report that cigarettes help them to relax and the intensity of smoking increases at times of stress. They also report that smoking has a tranquillizing effect when angry. These influences on subjective states do not tally with the neurochemical and physiological responses to nicotine.

Nicotine is a cholinergic agonist and so by acting as a brain stimulant is likely to enhance arousal. In this respect it differs from alcohol and the benzodiazepines. There is a secondary rise in plasma corticosteroids, an increase in central release of noradrenaline and in urinary catecholamine output. These changes are normally associated with the stress response so that the relaxing characteristics of nicotine present a paradox. A few theories attempting to resolve this conflict have been reviewed by Wesnes and Warburton (1983), though none fits all the experimental evidence satisfactorily. They argued that it is the action of nicotine on cholinergic pathways controlling attention that reduces stress by enabling individuals to concentrate more efficiently. Neurotic individuals, who comprise the majority of smokers, are helped by the drug to filter out distracting thoughts; this enables them to perform more effectively, increasing their self-confidence in the process.

Smokers tend to experience stress when trying to give up cigarettes.

For this reason games players and other athletes who smoke pre-competition need astute counselling in attempting to overcome the habit. This would be best done during non-critical periods of the week and the pre-match smoking could be replaced unobtrusively by behavioural techniques of relaxation. However, resort to smoking may be easily replaced by an increase in snacks between meals, leading to unwanted weight gain. This occurs because the appetite centre in the brain is released from the depressant effect that smoking has on it. This problem will be greatest in the casual recreationist whose energy expenditure during physical activity will generally be low.

Quite apart from the effects on health and on human performance, smoking may also have repercussions for sports injury, particularly under conditions of cold. An acute effect of smoking is peripheral vasoconstriction which decreases blood flow to the limbs. For this reason, the frost-bitten climber should avoid any temptation to smoke until after his recovery through hospitalization where alternative therapies are ensured.

Clearly, cigarette smoking has few advocates in sport and the sports sciences. Advertising of cigarettes is prohibited in some Scandinavian countries and top athletes are frequently prominent in anti-smoking campaigns. Smoking is rare among elite athletes, so that there are few models for youngsters taking up smoking to cite as examples. Those sports stars that do smoke might ultimately benefit from adopting alternative strategies to ease their troubled minds at times of stress.

5.7 Beta blockers

Sympathetic adrenergic nerve fibres are classified according to their alpha and beta receptors. Effects of these receptors are sometimes contradictory. In the blood vessels of muscle and skin, alpha-adrenergic receptors cause vasoconstriction, whereas beta receptors induce vasodilation. The beta receptors are further divided into $beta_1$ and $beta_2$ according to the responses to sympathomimetic drugs. Functions of $beta_1$ receptors include cardiac acceleration and increased myocardial contractility; $beta_2$ receptors cause bronchodilation and glycogenolysis. The action of these receptors is blocked by the activities of inhibitory drugs, the so-called beta blockers. These include, for example, atenolol, a cardioselective beta blocker with selectivity for beta-adrenoceptors; propranolol, which blocks both types of beta receptors, and labetalol which is a combined alpha and beta blocker. A more detailed description of sympathomimetic amines and their antagonists is given in Chapter 1.

Besides decreasing heart rate and myocardial contractility, the beta-blocking agents also reduce cardiac output, stroke volume and mean systemic arterial blood pressure. These effects explain the use of beta blockade in hypertension and in individuals with poor coronary health. Because of the effects on the circulation, beta blockade in clinical doses reduces maximal oxygen uptake and endurance time in normal individuals but increases maximal work capacity in patients with angina pectoris. At sub-maximal exercise levels a decrease in heart rate and contractility is balanced by a decrease in coronary blood flow and an increased duration of myocardial contraction. The fall in exercise heart rate is not matched by a corresponding drop in perceived exertion rating, so that the usual close correlation between these variables is dissociated by beta blockade.

The effects of beta blockers on metabolism have implications for the performance of sub-maximal exercise. By inhibiting the enzyme phosphorylase, beta blockade may decrease the rate of glycogenolysis in skeletal muscle. Breakdown of liver glycogen is also likely to be inhibited so that in sustained exercise blood glucose levels may decline. This fall is noted with propranolol but is not so evident with atenolol or metoprolol, two cardioselective beta blockers. Kaiser (1982) showed that jogging was markedly influenced only by propranolol at the low dose of 40 mg: at doses of 80 mg and above, atenolol had a similar adverse effect. Selective beta blockade inhibits lipolysis which may reduce the availability of free fatty acids as a substrate for prolonged exercise and cause an earlier onset of fatigue.

The effect of beta blockade on short-term high intensity performance was examined by Rusko et al. (1980). The subjects performed a range of anaerobic tasks after taking the beta blocker oxprenolol and results were compared with performances after being given an inert placebo. The drug had no effect on isometric strength of leg extension, vertical jumping and stair running. Total work output over 60 s on a cycle ergometer was reduced under the influence of the drug while peak lactates and heart rates were also decreased. It seems that the beta blocker caused a reduction in anaerobic capacity as well as in heart rate.

Use of beta blockers has implications for thermoregulation if exercise is conducted in the heat. Gordon et al. (1987) showed that a non-selective beta blocker (propranolol) produced greater sweating than did a beta$_1$-selective blocker (atenolol). In this study both drugs produced equivalent reductions in excercise tachycardia, a similar decrease in skin blood flow and a similar rise in rectal temperature. The authors suggested that beta$_1$-selective adrenoceptor blockers should be the preferred therapy during prolonged physical activity when adequate fluid replacement cannot be guaranteed. The findings indicated an increased need for persons treated with propranolol to stick to a strict fluid replacement regimen during sustained exercise.

Another consideration is whether the physiological adaptations to a fitness training programme are altered by the use of beta blockers. Propranolol, even in low doses of 80 mg daily, does blunt the effects of exercise training in normal individuals. At higher doses of 160–320 mg/day this impairment is more pronounced. The apparent mechanism is prevention of the normal peripheral circulatory and metabolic responses to exercise (Opie, 1986). Although beta blockade permits patients with angina to exercise more easily, the chronic effects of physical training in patients with ischaemic heart disease may still be attenuated. Indeed, Powles (1981) considered that the many physiological effects of beta blockade meant that for each patient there may be an optimal dosage. This optimal point is that at which adverse effects on the functioning of the left ventricle, the myocardial perfusion and metabolism did not outweigh the benefits associated with decreased heart rate.

Beta blockers cross the blood–brain barrier to varying extents depending on their lipid solubility (Table 5.5, Chapter 1); for example, propranolol does so to a greater degree than atenolol. Their anti-anxiety effect may not necessarily be centrally mediated. The suppression of cardiac activity which would result in a reduction in the afferent information from the heart may be the cause. Inhibition of the beta receptors, through which glycogenolysis is stimulated by adrenaline and lactic acid production increased, is an alternative mechanism. Low levels of lactic acid tend to be associated with a state of relaxation, free from anxiety. On balance, however, the evidence favours the interpretation that the anti-anxiety effects of these drugs are due to direct action within the central nervous system.

As beta-blocking agents are not addictive they tend to be preferred over the benzodiazepines and alcohol in combating anxiety. They attenuate emotional tachycardia, limb tremor and unpleasant manifestations of anxiety such as palmar sweating, pre-competition. High risk sports such as ski-jumping, motor-racing and bobsleighing provide especially suitable contexts for their use. Undesirable effects might be produced by beta blockers in athletes suffering from asthma and in individuals with reduced cardiac function.

The beta blockers have been banned by the International Shooting Union, as they are believed to be of potential use to marksmen in reducing anxiety before competitions and enhancing performance. Nevertheless, they were repeatedly used by many competitors in shooting events at the 1984 Olympic Games, being prescribed by team physicians for health reasons. Similar practices by top professional snooker players were disclosed at the 1987 World Championship. They are unlikely to be used in endurance events where the aerobic system is maximally or near-maximally taxed. They would have an ergogenic effect in the shooting discipline of the modern pentathlon, an event in which they have been allegedly used for a steadying influence before shooting.

The use of beta blockers in selected sports was reflected in the IOC Medical Commission's decision to only test for beta blockers in the biathlon, bobsled, figure skating, luge and ski jump competitions at the 1988 Winter Olympic Games in Calgary.

In the 1988 Summer Olympic Games in Seoul, it was the IOC Medical Commission's intention to only test for beta blockers in the archery, diving, equestrian, fencing, gymnastics, modern pentathlon, sailing, shooting and synchronized swimming events.

Studies of the effects of beta blockers on pistol shooters suggest that they are mainly of benefit to the less competent and less experienced shooters as well as those most anxious prior to competition (Siitonen, Sonck and Janne, 1977). A study of the British national pistol squad found that significant improvement in shooting scores was restricted to slow-fire events, the ergogenic effect being slightly greater for an 80 mg dose than for 40 mg of oxprenolol (Antal and Good, 1980). The effect of a 40 mg dose on rapid-fire scores was not significant. In a study of Belgian firearms specialists, the improvement in shooting performance resulting from a 40 mg dose of oxprenolol was matched by an effect of alcohol equivalent to a half pint (284 ml) of beer (S'Jongers *et al.*, 1987). There appeared to be a substantial placebo effect which applied equally to alcohol and beta blockers.

5.8 Overview

Stress and anxiety are inescapable corollaries of contemporary professional activities and participation in top-level sport. Indeed, a high degree of competitiveness seems to be a prerequisite for success in both spheres and those without the essential coping mechanisms fail to climb to the top of the ladder. The relationship between sport and anxiety is paradoxical in that sport as a recreational activity offers release from occupational cares, while at a highly competitive level it becomes a strong stressor. Indeed, exercise is effective therapy for highly anxious individuals, though this function was not central to the present topic. Nor was the role of behaviour modification strategies considered here, either as replacement for or complement to anti-anxiety drugs, although behavioural techniques have promise for the future in treating anxiety.

In the recent decade or so, sports officials and governing bodies in sport have assumed increasing responsibility for attempts to eliminate the use of drugs for ergogenic purposes. It is likely that the process of adding new pharmacological products to the list of banned substances will continue in spite of a running contest with those practitioners prepared to grasp at any means of improving their performances. The risks and benefits of anti-anxiety drugs as described, demonstrate that regulations for their use in sport must be set down with care and circumspection. Legislation must ensure that for the sport in question, participants especially prone to anxiety are not endangered by being deprived of their genuine prescriptions while at the same time allow fair competition to all entries.

5.9 References

Antal, L. C. and Good, C. S. (1980) Effects of oxprenolol on pistol shooting under stress. *The Practitioner*, **224**, 755-60.

Beckett, A. H. and Cowen, D. A. (1979) Misuse of drugs in sports. *Br. J. Sports Med.*, **12**, 185–94.

Blomqvist, G., Saltin, B. and Mitchell, J. (1970) Acute effects of ethanol ingestion on the response to submaximal and maximal exercise in man. *Circulation*, **62**, 463–70.

Corda, M. G., Concas, A. and Biggio, G. (1986) Stress and GABA receptors. In *Biochemical Aspects of Physical Exercise*, (eds G. Benzi, L. Packer and N. Siliprandi), Elsevier, Amsterdam, pp. 399–409.

Gordon, N. F., van Rensburg, T. P., Russell, H. M. S., Kielblock, A. J. and Myburgh, D. P. (1987) Effect of beta-adrenoceptor blockade and calcium antagonism, alone and in combination, on thermoregulation during pro-longed exercise. *Int. J. Sports Med.*, **8**, 1–5.

Hicks, J. A. (1976) An evaluation of the effect of sign brightness and the sign reading behaviour of alcohol impaired drivers. *Human Factors*, **18**, 45–52.

Ikai, M. and Steinhaus, A. H. (1961) Some factors modifying the expression of human strength. *J. App. Physiol.*, **16**, 157–61.

Juhlin-Dannfelt, A., Ahlberg, G., Hagenfelt, L., Jorfeldt, L. and Felig, P. (1977) Influence of ethanol on splanchnic and skeletal muscle substrate turnover during prolonged exercise in man. *Am. J. Physiol.*, **233**, E195–202.

Kaiser, P. (1982) Running performance as a function of the dose-response relationship to beta-adrenoceptor blockade. *Int. J. Sports Med.*, **3**, 29–32.

Luce, G. G. (1973) *Body Time: The Natural Rhythms of the Body*. Paladin, St Albans.

Opie, L. H. (1986) Biochemical and metabolic responses to beta-adrenergic blockade at rest and during exercise. In *Biochemical Aspects of Physical Exercise* (eds G. Benzi, L. Packer and N. Siliprandi), Elsevier, Amsterdam, pp. 423–33.

Powles, A. C. P. (1981) The effect of drugs on the cardiovascular response to exercise. *Med. and Sc. in Sports and Exer.*, **13**, 252–8.

Reilly, T. and Halliday, F. (1985) Influence of alcohol ingestion on tasks related to archery. *J. Hum. Ergol.*, **14**, 99–104.

Reilly, T., Lees, A., MacLaren, D. and Sanderson, F. H. (1985) Thrill and anxiety in adventure leisure parks. In *Proceedings of the Ergonomics Society's Conference*, (ed. D. Oborne), Taylor and Francis, London, pp. 210–14.

Rusko, H., Kantola, H., Luhtanen, P., Pulli, M., Videman, T. and Viitasalo, J. T. (1980) Effect of beta-blockade on performances requiring force, velocity, coordination and/or anaerobic metabolism. *J. Sports Med. Phys. Fit.*, **20**, 139–44.

Sanderson, F. H. (1981) The psychology of the injury-prone athlete. In *Sport Fitness and Sports Injuries*, (ed. T. Reilly), Faber and Faber, London, pp. 31–6.

Siitonen, L., Sonck, T. and Janne, J. (1977) Effect of beta-blockade on performance: use of beta-blockade in bowling and in shooting competitions. *J. Int. Med. Res.*, **5**, 359–66.

S'Jongers, J. J., Willain, P., Sierakowski, J., Vogelaere, P., Van Vlaenderen, G. and De Ruddel, M. (1978) Effect d'un placebo et de faibles doses d'un beta inhibiteur (oxprenolol) et d'alcool ethylique, sur la precision du tir sportif au pistolet. *Bruxelles-Medical*, **58**, 395–9.

Stepney, R. (1987) *Health and Lifestyle: A Review of a National Survey*. Health Promotion Research Trust, Cambridge.

Tong, J. E., Henderson, P. R. and Chipperfield, G. A. (1980) Effects of ethanol and tobacco on auditory vigilance performance. *Addictive Behaviours*, **5**, 153–8.

Wesnes, K. and Warburton, D. M. (1983) Stress and drugs. In *Stress and Fatigue in Human Performance*, (ed. R. Hockey), John Wiley, Chichester, pp. 203–43.

Wesnes, K. and Warburton, D. M. (1984) A comparison of temazepam and
  flurazepam in terms of sleep quality and residual changes in performance.
  Neuropsychobiology, 11, 255–99.
Wesnes, K. and Warburton, D. M. (1986) Effects of temazepam on sleep
  quality and subsequent mental efficiency under normal sleeping conditions
  and following delayed sleep onset. *Neuropsychobiology*, 15, 187–91.
Willett, W., Hennekens, C. H., Siegel, A. J., Adner, M. M. and Castelli, M. P.
  (1980) Alcohol consumption and high-density lipoprotein cholesterol in
  marathon runners. *N. Engl. J. Med.*, 303, 1159–61.

6

Future trends for drugs in sport

D. R. MOTTRAM

6.1 What is the purpose of sport?

There is, of course, no simple answer to this question. Sport serves different purposes for different people. At an amateur level it may simply be a recreational activity pursued for fun, excitement, or as a means of maintaining good health. At a more serious or professional level sport may be looked on as a means of employment for the individual or as a platform for commercialization for those in business. Either way sport does not exist without competitors. It is the complex motivating factors which drive the competitors that can make a sport what it is. These factors are themselves determined, to a large extent, by external influences. National pride, commercialism, media exposure and sponsorship will all affect the popularity of a particular sport which, in turn, determines the height to which a sportsman can attain notoriety or financial reward. The greater the incentives to succeed, the greater the temptation to use any method available to achieve that end.

Competition within sport is inevitably unfair. This may be due to the fact that a particular competitor is inherently physically better adapted to perform well in his chosen sport or that one competitor may have access to superior training equipment and schemes which are denied to another competitor. The rules of sport are designed to try to minimize these inequalities.

Frequently, sportsmen are either put under unacceptably severe external pressure or are no longer willing or able to submit to the demands of increased training schedules. Under these circumstances they turn to unfair means of attaining success. Drug misuse has unfortunately become one of the more popular forms of trying to beat the system.

6.2 What are the effects of drug misuse on sport?

To a greater or lesser degree, drug misuse affects individual sports, but more importantly, it is the individual drug taker who is more at risk. Perhaps it is unfair to imply that all sports are affected since there are many sports where drug taking does not take place. In other sports, cases of drug misuse are at best unreported thereby confining the problem to the individual rather than the sport as a whole. Adverse publicity regarding drug misuse must inevitably be detrimental to the sport and its organization. This will reduce the spectators' respect for the perpetrators and diminish the entertainment value of the sport. If the problem becomes endemic within a particular sport it may deter future participants from pursuing an interest in that sport.

With regard to the individual who misuses drugs to enhance performance, the effects may be both psychological and physical. Psychologically the athlete loses self respect and imposes a moral dilemma upon himself. Physically, the athlete is exposed to serious health hazards, particularly when involved in unsupervized drug taking. No drug is totally devoid of side effects and many possess potentially serious adverse properties which can lead to fatalities.

It is often assumed, quite incorrectly, that the drug taker will automatically win. The devastation at failing to attain superiority in his sport can lead the drug misuser to take higher and higher dose levels, with the consequent increase in the likelihood of toxicity. If research were to be carried out into the percentage of athletes who fail to win, despite their drug taking, this might in itself prove to be a significant deterrent to other drug takers.

A similar attitude of the drug-taking athlete is that of winning now, accepting the glory and frequently the financial rewards, and paying later in terms of ill-health. This would seem to be an extremely ill-advised course of action, particularly bearing in mind the severe long-term side effects of drugs such as anabolic steroids, and the potential dangers of drug habituation or addiction associated with other groups of drugs.

6.3 How should the problem of drug misuse in sport be tackled?

It must be accepted that a certain percentage of athletes will always be tempted by the promise of drug-induced enhancement of athletic performance. Therefore, any attempt to completely abolish drug misuse in sport is an unrealistic aim. There are, however, a number of measures that can be taken, and in some cases are being taken, to reduce the problem. These include preventative as well as punitive measures.

6.3.1 IMPROVED TESTING PROCEDURES

The ultimate deterrent for the drug taker is the fear of detection. The greater the risk of detection the lesser the likelihood of participating in drug taking.

With the advancement in technological sophistication the means by which drugs can be detected will continue to improve. However, success in drug detection is as much dependent upon the procedures for selection and sampling of the athlete as it is on instrumental analysis itself. Each sport organizing body must appreciate that drug misuse may be present, no matter how unlikely, within their sport. Sufficient measures need to be taken to ensure that competitors are tested not only at competitions but also, on a randomized basis, during training between events. Advice and recommendations for such testing is readily available from such bodies as the International Olympic Committee Medical Commission and through the European Antidoping Charter for Sport.

It is important that drug testing and detection methods should be consistent. This uniformity applies not only between sports, but also between nations, particularly concerning randomized testing between competitive events and on-site testing at national events. The European Antidoping Charter for Sport may in the future be extended to include other continents, with the possibility of a World Charter.

Finally, it is in everyone's interest to ensure that punishments previously laid down by the organizing body are actually implemented. Failure to carry out the punitive measures would only lead to contempt of the system and widespread abuse. On the other hand the athletes must feel that they have been treated justly and have received a fair hearing.

6.3.2 COLLABORATION

In discussing uniformity of drug-testing schemes in the section above, the importance of collaboration between organizing bodies was stressed. Collaboration must extend further than this. The problem of drug misuse in sport is such that discussions should take place at the highest level, between national governments. There are a number of ways in which governments can offer practical advice and help to sports organizations. It is encouraging to note that many national bodies now offer practical advice to sports organizations and to competitors themselves.

Encouragement should be given to ensure that sports organizations practice a uniform system of regulations and procedures for drug testing with an agreed list of banned substances. To this end, governments should assist in the funding of such activities particularly with respect to the high cost of drug testing laboratories.

In addition, governments could play an important role in promoting programmes of research into drug misuse in sport. This could be complemented by the implementation of educational programmes and campaigns aimed at participating athletes and, perhaps more importantly, potential athletes within schools and colleges.

6.3.3 RESEARCH

There are a number of misconceptions concerning drug misuse in sport. These are concerned with the potential benefit of drug taking, the capabilities of drug screening methods and the adverse effects of short- and long-term drug use. These misconceptions arise through ignorance on the part of the drug takers and their enablers. To a large extent this could be rectified through effective education programmes. However, to a significant degree, the basic information on which to derive an opinion on these matters is unavailable.

Research concerned with drugs in sport should centre on three main areas:

1. Drug effects on performance.
2. Attitudes towards drug taking.
3. Advances in analytical chemistry and biochemistry.

The first area of research poses significant pragmatic as well as ethical problems. It is extremely difficult to design suitable blind or double-blind trials, involving sufficient numbers of athletes, to derive scientifically accurate and acceptable data from which firm conclusions can be drawn. Ethically, one can criticize a study in which drugs are being administered to healthy human volunteers who are not in need of medication, particularly since the concentrations of drugs required to produce a meaningful comparison with the real situation are often far in excess of normal therapeutic levels. It is unfortunate that these constraints exist since it is exactly this type of unequivocal research that is needed to show the true value, or more likely the lack of value, of drug taking in sport.

A less controversial method of research involves attitude surveys of athletes themselves and of those closely associated with them. This type of research could reveal some very interesting results in terms of peoples' perceptions of drugs, their availability, effectiveness and side effects. The success of such a study would depend heavily on the nature of the questions asked of the respondent. Questions must be posed so as to receive an unequivocal answer. This would undoubtedly depend upon guaranteeing the anonymity for the respondent. Unfortunately, such research relies upon the integrity of those being questioned and too often the answer that is expected, rather than the truthful answer, is presented. The least contentious area of research is into developments of new techniques for drug detection and analysis. This type of research has proved extremely effective in the past and will continue to improve in the future.

Despite the demotivating factors associated with some areas of research it is important that studies should continue, thereby increasing the general breadth and depth of knowledge concerned with drug misuse in sport.

6.3.4 EDUCATION

In recent years, drugs have become more readily available for therapeutic and even recreational use. It should not, therefore, be surprising that some athletes have turned to these agents in an attempt to improve their performance in sport. Most of these athletes undoubtably realize that drugs cannot convert a mediocre sportsman into a top athlete. Nonetheless, they must consider that drug taking gives them that little bit extra, either physically or mentally, over their fellow competitors. They are probably intelligent enough to realize the harm which drugs can induce but either ignore the risk or decide to take a chance on it.

The listing of banned substances, the publication of rules against their use and the threats of disqualification against offenders will have had some deterent effect on athletes. However, others will see these measures as a challenge for which they must devise a system of evasion.

The real solution to the problem of drug misuse in sport lies in education, both for those not yet embarked in drug taking and for the rehabilitation of the misusers. Education must be a sustained long-term, process involving co-operation between various groups of individuals. Programmes of education should be devised and targeted to meet the different requirements of different audiences.

The organization for and dissemination of information should involve governments, national and local sports organizations, coaches and parents. Each of these groups required education themselves before the information is passed on to the athletes. In future, it should be possible for a greater number of athletes to accept personal responsibility for their behaviour towards themselves and their fellow competitors. With an effective programme of education it is to be hoped that athletes will compete without recourse to the use of drugs, thus re-emphasizing the ethical values of sport.

Index